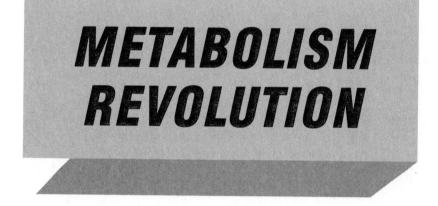

METABOLISM REVOLUTION

METABOLISM REVOLUTION

LOSE 14 POUNDS IN 14 DAYS AND KEEP IT OFF FOR LIFE

HAYLIE POMROY

WITH EVE ADAMSON

HARPER WAVE

An Imprint of HarperCollins*Publishers*

This book contains advice and information relating to health care. It should be used to supplement rather than replace the advice of your doctor or another trained health professional. If you know or suspect you have a health problem, it is recommended that you seek your physician's advice before embarking on any medical program or treatment. All efforts have been made to assure the accuracy of the information contained in this book as of the date of publication. This publisher and the author disclaim liability for any medical outcomes that may occur as a result of applying the methods suggested in this book.

FIRST EDITION

Library of Congress Cataloging-in-Publication Data

Names: Pomroy, Haylie, author.
Title: Metabolism revolution: lose 14 pounds in 14 days and keep it off for life / Haylie Pomroy with Eve Adamson.
Description: First edition. | New York, NY: Harper Wave, [2018] | Includes index.
Identifiers: LCCN 2017049820 (print) | LCCN 2017049127 (ebook) |
ISBN 9780062691637 (E-book) | ISBN 9780062691620 (print) |
Subjects: LCSH: Reducing diets—Recipes. | Weight loss. |
Metabolism—Regulation. | BISAC: HEALTH & FITNESS / Weight Loss. | HEALTH & FITNESS / Nutrition. | HEALTH & FITNESS / Healthy Living.
Classification: LCC RM222.2 (print) | LCC RM222.2 .P623 2018 (ebook) | DDC 613.2/5—dc23
LC record available at https://lccn.loc.gov/2017049820

18 19 20 21 22 LSC 10 9 8 7 6 5 4 3 2 1

I would like to dedicate this book to my sister-in-law Leilani Roh.
You are so bright and courageous.
Your light has led so many people to their journey.
Long after our work is done
I am so fortunate to get to walk beside you.

CONTENTS

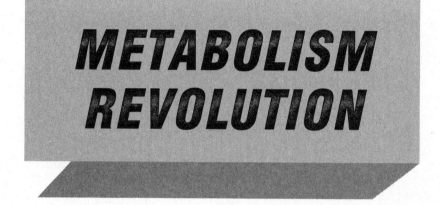

METABOLISM REVOLUTION

INTRODUCTION

As I was sitting down to write this, my sixth book on health, nutrition, and weight loss, I took a lot of time to reflect on my last twenty-two years of clinical practice. I thought about who comes to see me and what they have typically endured on their path to get here. Most of them land in my office after they've suffered years of body shaming and food struggles. Most of them have spent a lot of time and financial resources trying to achieve weight loss. Many of them are mad at their bodies. They are frustrated with their bellies. They are angry at their thighs. Yet here they are, sitting across from me—whether in an actual chair or virtually as they open the pages of one of my books—and telling me they will do *anything*. They will give up *anything*, because they are desperate to achieve the weight loss that keeps eluding them. Some come to me with well over 100 pounds to lose, and the very thought of that is overwhelming. Some have lost a lot of weight in the past but have gained it back and can't seem to summon the energy or the will to go through that weight loss process again. They want me to give them a boost—to help them find the necessary courage, to help them find hope that they really can lose it, and lose it for good.

Over the years, I have learned it is important to take a step back and look at the industry my clients have turned to for help, for resources, and for products. When I do that, I see how damaging constant dieting has been to them. It has slowed their metabolisms and dulled their motivation. It has disappointed them over and over again, and it has not kept them healthy. In many cases, it has sapped their health and vitality until they feel like they have almost none left. They have learned that starvation is necessary. They have learned that weight loss takes huge effort. They have learned that dieting comes at a steep price. Many of them believe that they just can't do it anymore. This is why we need a revolution.

I wrote this book in the spirit of revolutionizing the concept of what it means and what it feels like to lose weight. Although you may have learned otherwise, the truth is that weight loss doesn't have to be painful or boring. It doesn't have to take over your whole life. It can be easier than you think. And it can be fast. It can be effective. It can be delicious. And it can be good for your health. You don't have to sacrifice your skin, muscle tone, energy level, or satiety for weight loss. And you don't ever, ever have to starve. In fact, you *must not starve*. You can and should lose weight by eating food. It's the only way to work with your body's natural processes.

As my practice and my writing have evolved, along with my commitment and insatiable thirst to be a lifelong learner, I have watched my clients carefully to find out what they want and need from me. My flagship book, *The Fast Metabolism Diet*, helped millions of people repair their metabolisms and, in the process, lose up to 20 pounds in twenty-eight days. My other books, including *The Fast Metabolism Diet Cookbook*, *The Burn*, and *Fast Metabolism Food Rx*, have helped people tackle very specific weight loss and health barriers. Now, for the first time, because it is my constant quest to give you what you seek from me, I am unveiling my very latest, fastest-acting weight-loss plan yet. *Metabolism Revolution* can help you lose up to 14 pounds in just fourteen days by melting fat and stoking your metabolism to burn at an unprecedented rate. And it's all centered around food.

But super-accelerated weight loss is not all that is new about *Metabolism Revolution*. We are going to do some things I have never done with my community before. We are going to define your ideal body weight. We are going to rank the current state of your metabolic dysfunction (how far off you are from having a fast metabolism right now). We are going to define a body-specific intervention. And in fourteen days, we are going to revolutionize your metabolism so you can burn fat at a fast and furious rate.

If you are new to my work, welcome to my world. I am your nutritionist now, and I will take you under my wing and lead you through the amazing and wonderful world of eating for rapid weight loss and the maintenance of a fast metabolism while boosting your health and vitality so you will feel and look better than you have in perhaps a very long time. In fourteen days, you will lay down muscle, stimulate collagen production, burn fat aggressively, and realize outrageous weight loss without starvation or deprivation—up to a pound a day, day after day after day. You will look slimmer, feel tighter, be firmer and stronger, and have more luminous skin, shinier hair, and stronger nails. We are going to create meal maps together, and you will know exactly what you need to do every day. Everything is easier with clear instruction and constant support, and that is exactly what you will get from me. It won't be complicated. It won't be time-consuming. But it will work.

It's super simple—follow your meal map and choose your foods from the Metabolism Revolution Food List, or use the Metabolism Revolution Recipes customized for each meal map. You won't even have to think about it—fourteen days, and boom: rapid weight loss. You'll blow past historical set points, jump-start a large weight loss, or finally vanquish those last few stubborn pounds. It all depends on your Metabolic Intervention Score, which we will calculate together— once you know it, you will know your exact rapid weight loss strategy.

After that, in Part 2, I will help you decide what to do next. Do you have more weight to lose? You have effective options. Are you at your goal weight? Then you are going to need to know how to keep off that weight for life. The second half of this book contains a comprehensive 4 Life maintenance plan with a meal map for eating in a natural rhythm, a metabolism-stoking 4 Life Master Foods List, and answers to all your questions about the metabolic disruptors you will face living in our modern world. And when I say "4 life," I mean forever. I mean for when life happens to you, for when you need food-based therapeutic intervention, for when you go through menopause, for when you have a baby, for when you lose your job. In other words, you need to know how to sustain your weight loss *in real life*. Because as nice as it would be to have a personal chef or even a mom who still packs your lunch every day, or maybe to have every meal and snack delivered to your door, even in those über-supported situations, life happens. It happens to us all.

No matter who you are or what your circumstances, I always want you to know that there is power on your plate to lose weight, and there is power on your plate to keep it off for life. By the end of this book, you will have the tools you need for rapid weight loss success and steady and pleasurable weight maintenance. You'll be living the Fast Metabolism lifestyle with me, and I hope you will also join my active and inspirational community.

Even if losing weight fast in the past has not worked for you, this new plan promises to help you push past your set point and keep the weight off in ways that work for you, as an individual. There are many different reasons for weight gain, and many different paths to weight loss. In my other books, I target specific concerns, like thorough metabolic repair, weight loss plateaus for specific reasons, and chronic disease processes that can stall weight loss and impede health. Here I get more personal than I ever have before, with calculations that will customize your plan—so you can lose weight and regain health faster than ever. Rapid weight loss that also builds strength and health will not only help you feel better fast, but it will boost your confidence fast as you watch the number on the scale dropping every morning. The health piece happens simultaneously, as your nutrient-based weight loss triggers a cascade of positive metabolic changes that are real, proven, and documented. This rapid weight loss is both permanent and therapeutic. When you lose weight by stoking the metabolism with food, get ready to enjoy:

- A reduction in stress hormones
- Stabilized insulin and blood sugar levels
- Increased metabolic rate
- More efficient fat burning
- More energy, strength, and endurance
- An improved mood and greater self-confidence

After following this new plan, you will feel like you have flown across the country to see me in my private clinic without ever having to leave home. By combining the two elements my audiences say they love the most—fast weight loss and lots of amazingly delicious recipes—with a never-before-published plan that utilizes tactical protein gram rotations and proprietary food combinations to create significant weight loss without the crash-diet fallout, the *Metabolism Revolution* has everything you need to succeed. In the following pages, you will find:

- Customizable, easy-to-follow meal maps for everybody, exactly like my clients use.
- Nearly 100 delicious, lip-smacking, low-effort recipes, just the way my clients and community love them—all brand new and never before seen, and gorgeously photographed in stunning color. (And stay tuned for even more on our website.)
- Clear, doable food lists with foods you can find in any supermarket. Nothing hard to find or pricey—just real, whole food you recognize, in combinations you may never have thought to enjoy before.
- Options for every special diet. Vegetarian or vegan? Can do. Grain-free? No problem. Contented omnivore? Done and done.
- Foodies and kitchen-phobes will also find everything to meet their needs. I've seen it all, and my clients range from sophis-

ticated amateur chefs to those who would rather do just about anything than spend a day in the kitchen. I've got options for everyone.

- Once your weight is vanquished, you'll get a solid maintenance plan to keep you there, so you never have to worry about weight regain. You'll have all the tools to keep you exactly where you are. Or, if the need arises, to help you lose even more weight, whenever you are ready.

- All your questions answered, from newbie queries like how to eat in restaurants or what to eat on the road, to FMD (Fast Metabolism Diet) veteran questions about how to coordinate my various programs and live the FMD life long-term. You'll find out my latest and greatest metabolism tricks for occasional splurges, power snacking, exactly how and what to eat at parties and other social events, and much, much more.

You are my client now, and we are on this journey together. You have all the benefits of my clinical knowledge. You have all my resources. This book is in your hands, and we are a team. It's a done deal. You are about to revolutionize your metabolism. You are about to start burning fat for fuel at a furious pace. And you are about to start losing weight and feeling better. I can hardly wait to see what your body is going to do for you when we give it everything it needs. Welcome to the Revolution.

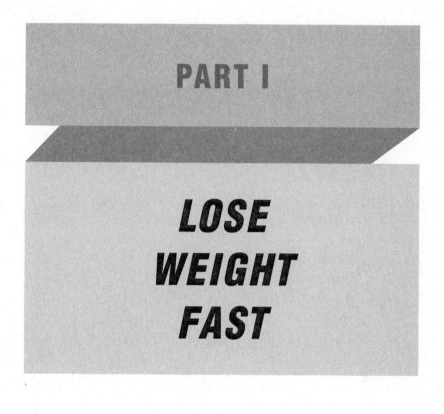

PART I

LOSE WEIGHT FAST

1

RAPID WEIGHT LOSS

That's it. We've all had enough. Conditions are unacceptable. It's time to stand up and say something. It's time to get up and do something—to put an end to oppression and systemic dysfunction. It's time to assert our rights, to change the whole system. *It's time for a revolution.*

A metabolism revolution, that is. If you are tired of trying diets that don't work or gaining back the weight you've lost, and you feel like you can't do it anymore, you need a metabolism revolution. If you keep cutting your food intake further and further but you still can't seem to get rid of the extra weight that makes you uncomfortable, you need a metabolism revolution. If you have scary risk factors for chronic disease, you need a metabolism revolution. If you think you're destined, or genetically predetermined, to be overweight and unhealthy, you need a metabolism revolution.

If your metabolism is not doing what you need it to do, you need to do something different. You need to shake it up. You need to change it out. You need to wake up your metabolism and get it burning hot and fast again. And there is only one way to do that.

I consider myself a kind of revolutionary—not just of the metabolism, but of a whole industry and mind-set that tries to invoke weight loss and health by taking away food. Ridiculous. I know, from more than twenty years of clinical experience and thousands of clients and readers who have lost literally millions of pounds, that taking away food to lose weight simply does not work. The reason I have been so successful is because I *never take food out of the equation*. I never take nutrients out of the equation. I am always looking to turn toward food, not away from food, as the way to speed up, heal, and repair the metabolism, and provide you with what your body needs to achieve rapid weight loss while also promoting glowing health. My methods are always nutrient-based and always metabolism-centric, because your metabolism is the secret to a healthy body that stays at a healthy weight.

So why do we keep believing the "fake news" that says dieting should be about deprivation, calorie restriction, or the elimination of major nutritious food groups? And even more relevant to this book, why do we keep believing that the only real way to lose weight permanently is to lose it slowly? This is the cultural message: Eat less, exercise more, and don't expect fast results. How uninspiring. How unmotivating. And according to the research, how ineffective. I know two things about weight loss, and I know them because I make them happen for my clients every day. What I know is that the best way to achieve real, meaningful, health-restoring, metabolism-stoking, life-changing weight loss is to:

1. Eat food—often more food than you are eating now; and
2. Lose weight as fast as possible.

Not only are we going to wake up your metabolism with food, but we are going to invoke rapid, permanent weight loss. Now *that* is what I call revolutionary. Traditional wisdom says you are supposed to lose weight slowly. That was the old belief, but thank goodness for progress. Now science is finally supporting what I have been telling my clients all along: You will get more weight loss, more motivation, more energy, and better health measures when you *lose weight fast*. As long as you know how to eat to maintain that weight loss, you are no more likely to regain that weight than someone who has lost it slowly. You may be even less likely to regain it. In other words, your rapid weight loss can be secure, stable, and permanent.

What Is Metabolism?

*M*etabolism is the process of converting food into fuel and using that fuel for energy. Your *metabolic rate* is the rate at which this happens. When it's slow, your body isn't efficient at converting food into fuel. The faster your metabolism, the better you can burn fat for fuel and convert nutrients into usable forms for building, repairing, healing, and energy production.

Although the metabolic process is complex, it also operates according to a few very simple natural laws, as real and unshakable as gravity:

LAW #1: The brain needs glucose to function. Glucose is brain fuel, and it only comes from food.

LAW #2: The body must store energy from food before it can be used. You can't instantaneously use the energy from an apple right after you eat it. You must convert it and store it first. This is a metabolic process, so your metabolism has to be working in order to store the energy from food.

LAW #3: The body must use stored energy to do anything, from growing to healing to moving. If it can't access the stored energy, it cannot function. If it doesn't have stored energy from food, it cannot function. If the metabolism isn't working well to access stored energy, then it will stay stored in your fat cells.

My entire practice and philosophy are based on these natural laws, which basically say *you need to eat food* to keep your metabolism at peak performance. You need to eat food so you have enough glucose to fuel the brain. You need to eat food so you can take in the micronutrients the metabolism needs to store energy. And you need to eat food to fuel the metabolism so it can access that stored energy, which you need to live your life.

In other words, to do anything, *including lose weight*, you need to eat food.

RAPID–WEIGHT LOSS BELIEFS

Let's look at that science and how it has evolved out of old ideas about what the pace of weight loss should be. Essentially, there are two conventional points of view about rapid weight loss:

Conventional Rapid Weight Loss View #1: *Rapid weight loss is good, at any cost.* For someone whose body weight severely and directly threatens their lives, drastic weight loss can be life-saving, but that doesn't apply to most people. If you embark upon a drastic weight loss regimen in a medical setting, you are likely to be given an extreme low-calorie diet, a liquid diet, or put on a fasting program. Or you might be given a more invasive intervention, which might be covered by insurance: Surgery to staple or tie the stomach so it is smaller. A wired-shut jaw to prevent overeating (or any eating). A prescription for pregnancy hormones, even though you are not pregnant. Many doctors advocate these methods because they do result in weight loss. They work. And isn't that better than being morbidly obese? Many medical professionals believe it is. The downside (other than the pain, the suffering, and the risk of long-term or permanent disability or even death) is that these methods involve literally starving a human being. On top of that, these radical methods have negative metabolic effects. When people lose weight in these ways, they will never again be able to eat the amount they ate before they became overweight. Their metabolisms are hobbled, and deprivation will be the name of the game for the rest of their days, or they risk gaining it all back—and having to go through the whole grueling, painful process again.

I cannot in good conscience believe that this kind of intervention is necessary for most people who need to lose weight. Because it is a non-nutrient-based method of rapid weight loss, it disrupts hormonal balance, encourages fat storage even at a very low-calorie intake, and often results in extreme hunger, low energy, aches and pains, saggy skin, hair loss, depression, and a general feeling of poor health. Need-less to say, that is not what I want for you.

Conventional Rapid Weight Loss View #2: Rapid weight loss doesn't last. Ac-cording to this belief, if you lose it fast, you will gain it back. Because aggressive methods so easily result in weight gain, this view says that to achieve lasting weight loss, "slow and steady wins the race." The people who advocate this approach believe that small, gradual, incre-mental lifestyle changes will supposedly help you lose ½ to 1 pound per week, a "safe" rate of weight loss, and they will be much less pu-nitive and much more pleasant. Sure, eating a tiny bit less and ex-ercising a tiny bit more is certainly more fun than major surgery or starvation. But there are serious problems with the effectiveness of this perspective.

Let's consider motivation. When you have 100 or more pounds to lose, or even 30 pounds to lose, then a slow-and-steady pace may seem not just frustrating but not worth the changes you have to make in your life. Why give up chocolate or cheeseburgers for a measly ½ pound weight loss per week? You'll spend *years* trying to lose 100 pounds at that rate. But even more problematic, what I see in my cli-ents is that with very slow lifestyle changes come very slow metabo-lism adjustments. Your metabolism likes to settle in at a comfortable spot, so as soon as you cut the chocolate, your metabolism adjusts to a chocolate-free life, so you are no longer inhabiting the same body that used to eat chocolate. Your body needs slightly fewer calories to stay where it is. You may lose a pound or two, but then that's all you get. You're going to have to give up something else if you want that weight loss to keep going. Suddenly, that ½ pound a week stops happening, and now even that 30-pound weight loss seems unattainable because nothing is happening at all. You may feel better if you are making better choices, but you may never see real, significant weight loss. And when weight loss slows or stalls completely, many people feel like they might as well give up and eat what they want to eat.

If you have ever tried either of these conventional methods, you may have found that they worked for a while or didn't work at all. But because they have been the only options out there, you may have continued to try different versions of them, over and over and over again.

I'm here to pull you off that crazy train. There is a third option. It's not part of the conventional view of rapid weight loss, but it is increasingly supported by the latest emerging science on how weight loss works.

Unconventional Rapid Weight Loss Belief: *Rapid weight loss driven by the strategic application of food and nutrients can increase health while dissolving fat and be permanent.* A rapid weight loss plan that feeds you rather than depriving you of food and nutrients can keep you from losing energy, experiencing extreme hunger, cannibalizing muscle, and sapping strength. When you use food to build muscle, burn fat, and increase the production of collagen and elastin—in other words, when you eat more, but choose the right foods at the right times—you can actually raise your metabolic rate, build strength, improve your skin tone, get more energy, and look incredible . . . all while giving you results you can measure, in record time.

This is the Metabolism Revolution. My clients don't have time for "slow and steady wins the race," and neither do you. They don't want all the negative side effects of extreme deprivation, and neither do you. They have lives to live, and they want to be able to enjoy food. I bet you do, too.

Science Geek Moment

Research backs up the notion that rapid weight loss is not more likely to result in weight regain, and is not more likely to repress metabolism than slow weight loss. As far back as 1984, research has demonstrated that in women who were very overweight, rapid weight loss resulted in a metabolism similar to that of women who were always lean.* Another study funded by the Australian National Health and Medical Research Council showed that "the rate of weight loss does not affect the proportion of weight regained within 144 weeks" and noted that "these findings are not consistent with present dietary guidelines which recommend gradual over rapid weight loss based on the belief that rapid weight loss is more quickly regained."† A University of Florida study concluded that "findings indicate both short- and long-term advantages to fast initial weight loss" and that "fast weight losers obtained greater weight reduction and long-term maintenance, and were not more susceptible to weight regain than gradual weight losers."‡ Finally, a *New England Journal of Medicine* study debunked several key myths about obesity, including demonstrating that it is *not true* that small, sustained changes in calorie intake or expenditure will lead to large long-term weight changes.§ It is also *not true* that setting realistic goals for weight loss is important because otherwise patients will become frustrated and lose less weight. So aim high. Let yourself embrace your ideal weight as a goal. The study also showed (like many others have) that it is not true that rapidly losing large amounts of weight is associated with poorer long-term outcomes than slower, more gradual weight loss.

---

*Well, SL, et al. "Resting metabolic rates of obese women after rapid weight loss." *J Clin Endocrinol Metabl*, 1984 Jul; 59(1): 41–4.

†Purcell, Katrina, et al. "The effect of rate of weight loss on long-term weight management: a randomized controlled trial." *The Lancet: Diabetes & Endocrinology*, December 2014; 2(12): 954–62.

‡Nackers, Lisa M., et al. "The Association Between Rate of Initial Weight Loss and Long-Term Success in Obesity Treatment: Does Slow and Steady Win the Race?" *Int J Behav Med*, September 2010; 17(3): 161–7.

§Casazza, Krista, et al. "Myths, Presumptions, and Facts About Obesity." *New England Journal of Medicine*, 2013; 368: 446–54.

Ultimately, you are the most important person in my equation. I have spent my career analyzing and experimenting with every weight loss option out there. It has taken me some time, but I am now confident—both from a research perspective and from what I see in front of me in my clinic every day—that nutrient-driven rapid weight loss is the best, the fastest, and the most supportive method of weight loss for vibrant health, high energy, and a fast metabolism.

You want to lose weight. I want you to lose weight. Forget all the distractions, the fads, and the extremes. Let's get back to food, and let's get this done.

SO YOU THINK YOU HAVE A SET POINT?

There is a belief that bodies have a "set point," or a weight at which they tend to settle or stabilize. This is true, in a way—there are times when the body pauses at a certain weight and seems to settle in and make itself comfortable. However, this is only a temporary condition, not a permanent one. When people come to see me in my office, they have often tried everything else they can think of, whether extreme or "slow and steady." They come to me because nothing else is working, but one of the most common things my clients tell me on our first visit is that they don't hold out too much hope because they believe, after years and years of dieting, that they have a "set point" and probably can't get below it. Some tell me they think they must have ruined their bodies, or permanently damaged their metabolisms, because they can't lose weight the way they used to. They think it is physically impossible for them to get back down to their pre-baby weight, or pre-injury weight, or peak athletic weight, or college weight. They ask me if they should just accept a higher weight. I hear things like, "I sure would love to weigh 145, but I can't get below 165 anymore, so maybe that's my set point?"

Most of these clients have lost weight and regained it repeatedly, and they always seem to get stuck. They say it feels like their bodies are fighting them, and that although it is a higher weight than they would like, or a weight at which they aren't yet comfortable, they're resigned to it. They look to me to confirm that yes, their expectations may be unrealistic because, yes, at a certain age, you have to weigh more. They think their set points have beaten them.

I say *nonsense*. You don't have a genetic set point or a post-baby set point or a menopause set point that you cannot change. Your metabolism is not preprogrammed with some special magic number that it will always go to by default.

Set points come from stress. When you experience significant stress, whether physical (an injury, a period of sickness, or time of extreme physical effort), emotional (any major life change that makes you feel insecure), lifestyle-based (lack of sleep, working the night shift, a difficult job), or from a major hormonal shift (puberty, pregnancy, menopause), your body adapts. This is a survival mechanism. Your current weight is always reflective of your current metabolic needs, and when you are under stress, your metabolism detects that "emergency" and starts storing fat. Your so-called set point is the point at which your body starts storing fat, and once more fat is on board, it changes the scenario.

Fat is not benign, inactive tissue. It is actually a secondary hormone-producing gland, which is why the body stores it. It is functional. If you are trying to burn fat for fuel or metabolize fat, your metabolism needs to feel that this is okay to do. It needs to be willing to give up that active hormone-producing gland. If you are under stress, your body won't want to take that risk, so it creates a sweet spot of safety—a set point below which it (temporarily) does not want to go. This is actually an amazing, genius-level strategy, and I, for one, applaud the human body for being so resourceful. But that doesn't help you when you really need to lose weight.

What that means is that if you are detecting a set point—if you have a weight you can't seem to get below—then something has to change. You need to convince your body that it is okay to release that stored fat. Starving yourself certainly won't do it. Stressing about your weight certainly won't do it. Hating your body definitely won't do it. But eating delicious food loaded with metabolism-fueling micronutrients? Practicing calming, relaxing behaviors? Moving your body gently and lovingly? Now we're talking.

Set points can have a strong gravitational pull, and when you move slowly over them, they can feel like the world's strongest magnet, always drawing you back to that number. Remember that you needed this internal force during times of stress, but anything that sends a signal to your body that you are doing awesome, thank you very much, and the emergency is over, will blow through that set point like it's yesterday's news—which it is. Score another point for nutrient-based weight loss.

Food is the source for the fuel you need to build and maintain a healthy human body. All your metabolic processes, including the conversion of stored energy, are nutrient dependent. If you aren't eating enough, such as during a crash diet or while fasting, you can't give your body the nutrients it needs to convert stored energy to usable energy. Carbohydrates feed your brain and create energy. Protein builds your structure. Fat facilitates hormone production and absorption. Vitamins and minerals help keep your metabolic pathways functioning. You need it all, and you're going to get it all. Food is going to make things happen for you . . . and it's going to happen fast. I've shepherded hundreds of clients through this process, and they've blown past their historical set points and lost weight faster than they ever could have imagined, without doing anything that felt extreme. Let's meet some of them.

Janet and Her Health Risk Problem

Janet came to me after losing 60 pounds. She needed to lose almost 60 pounds more, but she had run out of steam, had gone off her program, and was no longer motivated. She was burned-out by deprivation. She was tired—not just tired of dieting, but overwhelmed by chronic fatigue due to her poor health.

Janet initially decided to lose weight because her doctor warned her that she had many risk factors for heart disease, and although she had some improvement with her initial weight loss, she still had measurable issues—high cholesterol, high blood pressure, and high blood sugar. We both agreed that the weight had to come off, once and for all, so she never had to worry about it again, but because she didn't feel good, Janet found it very hard to make herself do what she knew she had to do. She admitted that she had slipped back into her junk food habit, was eating too much sugar, and hardly ever ate vegetables anymore. To her, it seemed like a long and ponderous road to health, when all she wanted to do was curl up with some yummy food and watch television. So I asked her, "Can you give me fourteen days?" We would get this done fast. I told her I could get 14 pounds off her in fourteen days. Once the scale was on the move again and she was feeling more energy and motivation, I knew she would feel better and have more energy for a longer-term commitment to a more health-promoting lifestyle. Janet decided that she could summon up the energy for two weeks of organized eating, so I laid out fourteen days for her, showing her every single thing she would have to do. No thinking involved. Hardly any food prep. I told her it would be easy, the food would be simple but satisfying, and she would finally start losing weight again . . . and fast.

Sure enough, fourteen days later, Janet was actually down 15 pounds. She told me she had more energy than she had had in years, and she couldn't believe how quickly it had all happened. She decided to do another round of the Metabolism Revolution plan, and when I spoke to her recently, she was down another 10 pounds, her cholesterol was almost back in normal range, her blood sugar was all the way back in normal range, and her blood pressure was heading steadily downward, too. I predict she will be at her goal weight very soon.

What Makes Weight Loss Slow to a Grinding Halt?

Stress comes in many forms: a physically toxic environment (like pollution and chemicals in food), an emotionally toxic environment (like a dysfunctional relationship or a defeating job), or a life-changing event (from a wedding to a divorce, a move or a job change or the loss of a friend or family member). Stress can be acute, like getting into a car accident or breaking your leg. And stress can be chronic, for example, if you travel all the time or you are a caregiver or your job is highly demanding but not highly rewarding. Even dieting—especially crash dieting, fasting, and very-low-calorie diets—is extremely stressful to the body. Stress also puts you at risk of gaining back all the weight you worked so hard to lose, because stress predisposes the body to excessive fat storage, because the body attempts to rescue us from these exposures by sealing away toxins in fat cells and refusing to let them out.

Lucy and Her Supposedly Immovable Set Point

When Lucy came to my office for the first time, she told me she didn't care about "looking like a model." She looked like she was of a pretty average weight to my eyes, with cute curves and a bubbly personality. She told me that she wanted to lose 12 pounds because she knew from past experience that she was about 12 pounds above the weight that made her feel like her best self. "I still want these curves," she said, slapping her hips, "but I'm not quite where I feel my best, and no matter what I do, I can't get back down there."

The problem was that every time she went on a diet, she was only able to get down to about 168 pounds or, at the lowest, 165 pounds. She could never get below that number. She had given up and drifted back up to 170 pounds. She brought in a printout of a research study about set points, dropped it on my desk, and said, "Well, I guess 165 is as good as it gets for me."

I explained to Lucy that set points are temporary roadblocks to weight loss, erected by the metabolism in response to stress. When she thought about it, Lucy said she remembered that she had gained about 30 pounds when she went away to college, and had never been able to lose it again. We decided that the Metabolism Revolution was just the fast-acting intervention Lucy needed to prove to herself that her set point was not a permanent condition.

Sure enough, Lucy plowed right past her supposed set point, and by the end of fourteen days, she weighed 159 pounds. She was thrilled, and best of all, she finally felt comfortable in her body.

Kelly and Her Impatience Problem

A client of mine named Kelly wanted to lose 70 pounds, and I agreed that this was a good goal to put her into a healthy weight range for her height. She had been working at weight loss, with a weight loss plan and group meetings, following that plan's recommended slow-but-steady weight loss goal of 1 to 2 pounds per week. Everybody was happy for her. According to her current program, she was a diet success. She was indeed losing approximately a pound a week, most of the time. However, because she had so much weight to lose, she was getting frustrated and impatient. She felt like it would take forever to see any real progress. She told me, "You know, I never get a real payoff. I never lose enough weight in a week that I can't undo it all in one night of 'off-plan' eating like going to a restaurant or a party. Then it's like I never lost any weight at all. At this rate, I won't be close to my goal weight for over a year, and I don't know if I can sustain this that long. How is this worth all the effort I'm putting in?"

Kelly didn't really believe she would ever reach her goal, and was beginning to think that life at a healthy weight would never be possible for her. I told her that a more rapid weight loss pace would be much more motivating for her and give her the response her body deserved. I showed her a fourteen-day plan that would evoke significant weight loss in a healthy way—½ to 1 pound *per day*—and we agreed that when this really worked, she would be reinspired by her body and back in awe of what she was capable of doing. I wanted Kelly to get back to loving the way she felt when her body was rapidly burning fat for fuel.

Kelly switched from her group plan to Metabolism Revolution, and fourteen days later, she couldn't believe the difference. "I finally feel like something is happening." she said. "My whole body feels different— stronger, more energetic. This is awesome." Kelly did miss the community support of her previous program, so I introduced her to our gold member program (you can visit, too, at https://hayliepomroy.com /become-a-member/) and our Facebook page (www.facebook.com /hayliepomroy/), and she quickly made new friends and loved all the before-and-after pictures and inspirational stories as well as the encouragement she found. In fourteen days, Kelly had lost exactly 14 pounds, but even better, she had gained motivation and was much more optimistic about reaching her goal weight.

Laura and Her Fertility Problem

Laura landed in my office because her doctor had referred her to a very famous weight loss doctor, known for his starvation plans, who happened to have an office in my neighborhood but also happened to be on vacation. I was next on the list, so he sent her to me. Laura was not having a good response to fertility-stimulating drugs, and her doctor had seen some information about rapid weight loss and how it can alter hormone receptivity. He told Laura, "I don't care how you do it, but I need you to be ten pounds lighter over the next four weeks." When Laura told me this, I told her, "We can do it in two. Let's map out your next fourteen days, let's get these ten pounds off, and let's get you pregnant."

Laura loved the easy, nutrient-dense plan. She told me she felt like it was not only helping with her weight loss and energy, but that she was getting her body totally prepped for her future baby. Six months later, Laura was pregnant, and ended up delivering a healthy baby girl.

Michael and His Cholesterol Problem

I have plenty of male clients, too, so let's talk about Michael. When Michael initially came to see me, he weighed 237 pounds. I put him on one of my longer-term weight loss plans and we got him down to about 195 pounds over a period of three to six months. He felt really good at 195. He was on Lipitor (a cholesterol-lowering drug), and with this weight loss, he was able to reduce his daily dosage from 40 mg to 10 mg.

When he came to my office again three years later, looking handsome in a dapper suit, I remarked on how good he looked. "Not good enough," he said. He had successfully maintained his weight right about 195 pounds since I'd last seen him and had recently asked his doctor about getting off Lipitor completely. But his doctor said he would only allow it if Michael could get down to 185 pounds. He had already experienced great relief from his breathing problems and knee pain at 195 pounds, but now he had a new motivation to start losing weight again. Metabolism Revolution was the perfect plan to get rid of those last 10 pounds. We easily got him to 185 by the end of two weeks, and his doctor took him off Lipitor entirely. Michael's cholesterol and blood sugar are now in the normal range without the help of medication, and he feels even better than he did before. Two years later, he is still happily maintaining at 185 pounds.

WHAT RAPID WEIGHT LOSS CAN DO FOR YOU

Just the other day, I was out fishing with my kids, and my line got stuck under some rocks. I was pulling and pulling and reeling and pulling, and I thought I was going to break the line. Then one of the boat hands came around by the dock and said, "You have to jerk it loose." He gave it a swift jerk, and the line was dislodged. "Huh," I said. "That was easy."

This is what the Metabolism Revolution can do for you. Sometimes you are pulling and pulling and reeling and pulling to lose weight the way you think you are supposed to lose weight, and it isn't getting you anywhere. You are stuck and frustrated, but all you need to do is change the angle and give it a jerk. Whether you are a yo-yo dieter or a slow-and-steady dieter or someone who feels like they should be a dieter or someday could be a dieter, we all have a common goal. We want to get the scale to move. This is what you want, what you need, what your doctor is telling you you need. Let's get you some results quickly so you can feel good about the effort you're putting in. Let's get you feeling good about your body and the way it performs in response to your efforts.

Why did I choose this plan for Michael? Because he was ready to take his health to the next level. Why did I choose this plan for Janet? Because she wanted to beat chronic disease and live her life, active and worry-free. Why did I choose this plan for Lucy? Because she needed to take down her supposed set point once and for all. Why did I choose this diet for Kelly? Because slow and steady was too slow for her. Why did I choose this plan for Laura? Because she needed to jump-start her hormones. Now you and I are going to revolutionize *your* metabolism. We are going to get you unstuck, get that fat to move, and unleash the energy you need. We're going to figure out exactly where you want to be, weight-wise, and what your body needs to get that done. Then we are going to create the perfect plan to get the weight off and take you through the process of keeping it off for life.

The bottom line is that slow-and-steady weight loss is 1 to 2 pounds per week, and that is not going to accomplish all the amazing things you want for your body and your life. Fast weight loss is $\frac{1}{2}$ to 1 pound *per day*, but it is so much more. It is a metabolism reboot. It is a hormonal system makeover. It is a whole new life. Fast weight loss is what you can and will accomplish with the Metabolism Revolution. All you have to do for proof is go to my website (hayliepomroy.com) or our Facebook community (www.facebook.com/hayliepomroy/), and you will see story after amazing story, before-and-after pictures that will blow your mind, and real people talking about how rapid weight loss (whether they call it that or not) has completely transformed their lives for the better.

If you are a little freaked out right now by the possibilities of this promise, spend a little time looking at those testimonials. You can do this. I've taken thousands of people through this process, and it works. Now it's your turn to let it work for you.

2

METABOLIC DYSFUNCTION AND IDEAL BODY WEIGHT

What you weigh and how well your metabolism is working are not always directly correlated, but in most cases, excess fat storage is one of the most obvious signs of metabolic dysfunction. So let's talk weight. What do you think you should weigh? Maybe you have a number in mind. Or maybe you have two numbers in mind—the number you would really like to weigh, and the number you think is probably as low as you're going to get at this stage in your life. Maybe that first number, the number you would really like to weigh, is what you weighed at a time in your life when you felt really good—or maybe you know you used to weigh that much, but you honestly can't remember because it's been so long. Maybe that second number, your "resignation number," is your current weight, or the weight you typically achieve when you go on a diet, although you go back above it again as soon as you go off the diet.

We put so much emotion and worry into those numbers. But what really determines them is metabolism. Let's spend a little bit of time considering how that works, so we know what we need to do in your body to make the number you want happen for you. Because yes . . . you can make that number happen.

Ideal Weight Calculator

What is your ideal weight? Is it the number you think it is, or is it something completely different? Ideally, I like my clients to have an ideal weight *range*, because weight fluctuates from day to day for many reasons. For our metabolic dysfunction calculation, however, you will need a specific number, so let's figure out a range as well as a target number.*

MINIMUM IDEAL WEIGHT

100 pounds +/- 5 pounds for every inch over/under 5 feet = minimum ideal weight

Fill in your numbers based on the above calculation:

100 pounds +/- ▮▮▮▮▮▮▮▮▮▮ **=**

5 pounds for every inch over/under 5 feet

▮▮▮▮▮▮▮

minimum ideal weight

MAXIMUM IDEAL WEIGHT

If you are 5 feet 8 inches or shorter:

100 pounds +/- 12 pounds for every inch over/under 5 feet = maximum ideal weight

Fill in your numbers based on the above calculation:

100 pounds +/- ▮▮▮▮▮▮▮▮▮ **=**

12 pounds for every inch over/under 5 feet

▮▮▮▮▮▮▮

maximum ideal weight

---

* Special note for people 5 feet tall and under: Every pound is a larger percentage of your body weight than a taller person, so your weight range will be less. If you are 5 feet tall, ideally you should fluctuate between 95 and 105 pounds. If you are shorter than 5 feet, you can subtract 5 pounds for every inch below 5 feet, but I do not recommend weighing less than 90 pounds, no matter how short you are.

If you are 5 feet 9 inches or taller:

100 pounds + 10 pounds for every inch over 5 feet = maximum ideal weight

Fill in your numbers based on the above calculation:

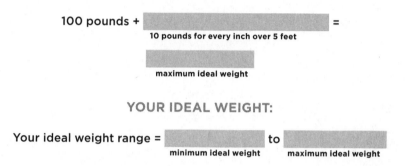

YOUR IDEAL WEIGHT:

Your ideal weight range =   to
                          minimum ideal weight   maximum ideal weight

Finally, your ideal weight is somewhere in the range between your calculated minimum and maximum. Choose a number in that range that feels comfortable for you.

Your ideal weight =
                    any number you choose within the above range, as a goal

Why Not Use the BMI?

There are many ways to determine ideal weight, and a popular method health professionals like is the body mass index (BMI) system. I am not in favor of it because the BMI was originally developed to look at generalized health trends. It was never intended to assess the weight of individual people, and it does not work well for very muscular, very tall, or very short people.

Not Your Idea of Your Ideal Weight?

Sometimes, my clients want to challenge me about their weight range. They think the low end is too high, or the high end is too low. They often have the wrong idea about what people actually weigh, or what people should weigh—or they have a picture in their head, maybe based on someone they know or a celebrity or something someone told them.

Trust me, if you knew what real people really weigh (including celebrities), you would probably not feel so bad about your own weight, but if you really do believe you should weigh less than your calculated minimum, or more than your calculated maximum, I recommend getting some personal nutrition counseling to do this safely, especially if you want to weigh less than your minimum. There are significant health risks to not having enough structure or enough nutrients to sustain your structure. If you are going to alter your structure significantly, you must protect the muscle and the bone through measuring and monitoring by a health professional. So, for example, if you are 5 feet 10 inches tall and you want to weigh less than 150 pounds, I recommend an in-depth physical before I support your desire to be lighter than that. I want you to be healthy, above all.

WHY WE GAIN EXCESS WEIGHT

When we gain weight, our bodies store more energy than they burn. You might be saying, "Duh, Haylie. Everybody knows that." However, let's take a step back and look at what that really means. "Our bodies store more energy than they burn" is not the same as saying "Eat less, exercise more." There are many metabolic forces at work at any given moment in your life that determine exactly where and why your body decides to store energy, and when and why your body decides to burn energy.

If you got a group of your friends and family together, and everybody ate a single doughnut, each person in that group would use that energy a little bit differently. Some might burn it off almost immediately. Others might store every bit of that doughnut directly in their fat cells. Most are probably somewhere in between, all along a complex spectrum of storing and burning, and the difference is metabolism. Everyone has a very particular metabolic process going on inside them, and it is a process that you can largely control, based on what you do. You could be the super-burner, or you could be the super-storer, or you could store some and burn some.

Have you ever wondered why your body would decide to store fat when you clearly have plenty of fat stores already on deck? Have you ever wondered why your body became so resistant to weight loss, even though your doctor told you that losing weight would improve your health? Why would a smart body choose to hold on to excess weight? There is always a reason.

If it has become easier for you to gain weight than to lose weight, your body is in some state of metabolic dysfunction. I define *metabolic dysfunction* as the inability to effectively burn fat for fuel and the overdeveloped tendency to store fat in unwanted and undesirable locations on or around the body. But your metabolism didn't get that way randomly. It isn't working as well as it could because that is how your body is responding to something in your environment. Metabolism dysfunction is a survival mechanism. There is a "why" behind what is going on with you. Maybe your body isn't getting the micronutrients it needs, so it has to shut down or slow down some systems in order to keep functioning. Maybe you have been under stress, and your body was storing fat for an emergency. Maybe you will never know the reason, but trust me when I tell you that there is a reason. Your body is not stupid, and your body is not capricious. It does its best for you in every moment of living. Now it's your turn to do your best for your body.

But before we can know for sure what is best for your individual body, we need to assess your current level of metabolic dysfunction. How far off the path have you gone? Where are you right now? This will help us determine what you need to get your metabolism back to full function and robust working order.

PRIMARY SIGNS OF METABOLIC DYSFUNCTION

If you are in a state of metabolic dysfunction, your body is already trying to tell you that. Check the box next to any questions to which you can answer YES:

I.

❑ Have you noticed the sudden appearance of fat where you never had fat before, like belly fat, fat along the bra strap line, protruding hip fat, or fat under the arms or behind the knees?

❑ Are you feeling joint or muscle pain not related to an injury, especially all over, or on both sides of your body at the same time?

❑ Have you noticed that your energy is lower than usual?

❑ Have you been experiencing mood swings you can't seem to control very well, like sudden irritability, crying, anger, or sadness?

❑ Are you having trouble getting to sleep, or are you waking up in the middle of the night and not able to fall back to sleep easily?

❑ Are you experiencing disturbing menopausal symptoms like hot flashes, hair loss or gain, PMS, irregular menstrual cycles, menstrual migraines, or lack of libido?

❑ Do you feel cold all the time even when other people don't, or are your hands or feet always cold?

❑ Do you think you get too easily stressed, out of proportion to the situation?

II.

❑ Has your doctor told you that you have abnormal results on lab tests?
  ❑ Vitamin D deficiency
  ❑ Elevated total cholesterol
  ❑ Low HDL cholesterol

❑ High LDL cholesterol
❑ Elevated hemoglobin A1C
❑ Elevated fasting blood sugar
❑ Elevated C-reactive protein (CRP) or other inflammatory markers

III.

❑ Have you received any of the following diagnoses from your doctor?
❑ Polycystic ovarian syndrome
❑ Endometriosis and/or adenomyosis
❑ Hypothyroidism
❑ Autoimmune disease
❑ Diabetes or metabolic syndrome

If you checked three or more of the items on the first list, two or more items on the list of lab tests, or even one item on the diagnosis list, I want you to know that your condition is not normal. Your metabolism is not working like it should, and it is calling out to you for something. Don't be mad at your body. Be curious. Listen. And most important, don't be okay with the situation. Metabolic dysfunction is not something that "just happens" with age or overeating or menopause or whatever you have been blaming your weight gain and low energy on recently. There are plenty of healthy people with fast-burning metabolisms who are older, or who eat a lot, or who are in menopause. You probably know them. And you can be one of them. You need to repair your metabolism . . . and fast.

THE SLOW METABOLISM SPIRAL

When I talk about metabolic dysfunction, what I mean is that your metabolism is slow. The degree of metabolic dysfunction directly correlates to the rate of your metabolism. Remember that metabolism is the rate at which you convert the energy from food into the processes your body needs to live life. Rate is about speed. The higher the metabolic dysfunction, the slower the metabolism, and the healthier the metabolism, the faster it burns. This is why I always talk about achieving a fast metabolism—a fast metabolism is a strong and healthy metabolism.

Now let's think about what a slow or dysfunctional metabolism looks like in your body. When your metabolism is dysfunctional, a few very important things happen that directly impact your weight and health:

1. *You prioritize burning simple carbohydrates.* Let's say you come home after a long day at work and you are exhausted, and then somebody in your family says, "What's for dinner?" When you are exhausted, do you want to cook something elaborate, or do you want to order something to be delivered? Delivery is easier, of course. So is carbohydrate metabolism. When you are exhausted and stressed, your body isn't going to hunt around for proteins and fats to convert and metabolize. Way too much work. Proteins and fats take a lot of energy to break down into micronutrients. They provide slow, steady fuel, which is great in theory, but your metabolism is basically throwing up its hands and saying, "Let's just order pizza!" Simple carbs break down quickly, providing fast energy, even if it doesn't last long. This is why you are more likely to crave carbs when you are stressed or tired. (The next time that happens, imagine your body metaphorically ordering pizza while the veggies and fruit rot in the crisper.)

2. *You prioritize fat storage.* A dysfunctional metabolism prioritizes fat storage because long-term survival is more important than short-term looking-good-in-skinny-jeans. This often happens to people on calorie-restrictive diets, but it also happens when people are under stress. To use food for energy, the metabolism has to convert it for storage, then use those stores for function-

ing. A dysfunctional metabolism tends to stuff every incoming calorie into fat storage, like a squirrel stocking a tree with acorns for the long winter. If your body thinks winter is coming, then it doesn't matter what you eat—a candy bar, an apple, even celery and lettuce. It's all going into the tree.

3. *You aren't extracting enough micronutrients from food.* Imagine you are really good at doing brain surgery. You are the best surgeon in the country. But you wake up one morning with a horrible case of the flu. Or you stay up all night and now you can barely keep your eyes open. This is no time to perform brain surgery. Even if you know how to do it, that doesn't mean you are in a condition to do it. A dysfunctional metabolism is much the same. Your body knows how to extract micronutrients from food, but the many complex biochemical processes required to do this are not working very well—they are nodding off because they are exhausted. That means all the things you want happening in your body, like burning fat for fuel and hormone production and utilization, all depend on micronutrients, and you aren't accessing them.

When you can't extract those micronutrients, your metabolic dysfunction gets more severe because it needs those micronutrients to stay awake and get to work. Then you get stuck in a vicious circle of nutrient deprivation, resulting in even worse metabolic dysfunction. Even the most nutrient-rich foods won't help you if you don't have the capacity to break them down.

If you are experiencing metabolic dysfunction and you haven't been able to achieve the weight you want, it's not your fault. It's not a lack of willpower. Intense cravings are not a sign of weakness. You are gaining weight because your body is telling you to eat more due to its perceived lack of nutrition, while aggressively storing energy as fat to guard against further nutrient deficiency. But at the same time, it is not extracting micronutrients that your metabolism needs to function properly, which is what has led your body to feel you aren't getting nourished in the first place. Theoretically, this is a heroic effort by your body, but realistically, it's a vicious and negative spiral of metabolic dysfunction. As that dysfunction increases and more metabolic pathways go down, your body continues to compensate to protect itself from perceived starvation, but the price you pay is weight gain, low energy, or even chronic disease.

If this sounds like you, then we need to turn things around. We need to reverse that spiral so we can repair your metabolism and get it burning hot and fast again. That means we have to:

1. Replenish your energy stores, so your body can summon up the energy to digest protein, fat, and complex carbs, as well as simple carbs.
2. Convince your body that there is no emergency and it does not need to continue storing all the energy you eat in the fat cells.
3. After the body is calmed and has energy again, encourage micronutrient extraction with the strategic use and timing of nutrient-dense foods.

CALCULATING YOUR METABOLIC DYSFUNCTION RANK

I know you are ready to start losing weight now, and I know you want to get it off quickly. You might be inclined to say, "Haylie, just tell me what to eat." My clients say this to me all the time—"I've got to get this weight off. I'll do whatever you say. Tell me what to eat." My response to you, as it is to them, is that we've got to get to know you and understand your body together before we can have the outrageous success you desire. When we know what your body is doing right now, I will have a much better idea of how to get that weight off you, fast.

In general, I find that my clients who want to lose weight fall into one of three categories:

- The Magic Zone, where you don't have much to lose but your weight feels stable, so it is difficult to get those last few pounds off.
- The Unstable Zone, where weight loss is relatively easy but so is weight regain.
- The Weight Loss Resistance Zone, where you've gained a lot but you can't seem to lose it because it feels like your "new normal."

I'll tell you more about these zones when you figure out where you are. To discover which zone you are in right now, let's calculate your Metabolic Dysfunction Score. You will need your ideal weight goal from page 29 for this next calculation.

Metabolic Dysfunction Rank

STEP ONE:

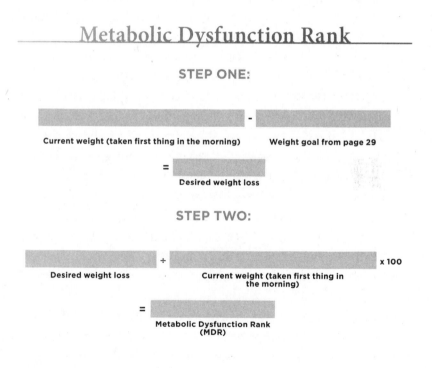

Current weight (taken first thing in the morning)   Weight goal from page 29

Desired weight loss

STEP TWO:

Desired weight loss   Current weight (taken first thing in the morning)   x 100

Metabolic Dysfunction Rank
(MDR)

METABOLIC DYSFUNCTION RANK: WHAT DOES IT TELL ME?

Your MDR will fall into one of three categories:

1. *2 to 7: Magic Zone.* This is the zone where your body becomes stable and creates homeostasis. It feels comfortable here, even when you still aren't quite to your ideal weight. This is where you can eat a lot and party once or twice a week and still stay at the same stable weight. This is the range where your muscle to fat to bone ratio is conducive to a healthy metabolism—that's why I call it the Magic Zone. But it doesn't mean you are quite where you want to be. This stability is why those last 3 to 5 pounds can feel so stubborn . . . but don't worry, we will get them off.

2. *8 to 15: Unstable Zone.* Your metabolism is less stable in this zone, so when you are here after losing a lot of weight, you probably have a sense of anxiety about it. You are afraid the weight will come back before you get all the way to your goal. That is understandable, because this is the tipping-point zone. Your body is easily influenced in either direction. People who yo-yo diet a lot tend to do so within this range, chasing a number up and down on the scale. When I have clients in this zone, I advise them to put their heads down and don't look up for fourteen days, until we get them into the Magic Zone, where they will feel more stable.

3. *Any number greater than 15: Weight Loss Resistance Zone.* When you are in this zone, your body favors the metabolic pathways for weight gain over the metabolic pathways for weight loss, making weight loss more difficult. This zone contains a lot of historical set points—numbers my clients tell me they haven't been able to get below since having their first child, for example. The goal for people in this zone is to change the metabolic environ-

ment swiftly and dramatically, to blow past those historical set points and into a more active weight loss state.

What zone are you in right now? This will change over time as you lose weight and get healthier, but what concerns us is where you are today. Knowing this will help us recognize what kind of challenges you have ahead, but no matter where you land, the Metabolism Revolution will be customized to get your weight moving in the right direction and end your weight loss struggles for good. Now it's time to define the plan that is going to get you out of the place you are stuck in right now. It's time for a metabolic intervention.

3

CUSTOMIZING YOUR METABOLIC INTERVENTION

Now that we know what kind of challenge we have ahead of us, it's time to create a customized eating plan that will pull you right out of your metabolic dysfunction. To accomplish that goal, we will calculate your Metabolic Intervention Score (MIS), which will direct you to one of my three customized meal maps. Your meal map will advise you exactly what food categories to eat and in what amounts, and will also give you a customized exercise plan designed to burn fat most efficiently for your MIS. As I explained in the introduction, rapid weight loss is effective only when the plan is nutrient-based, targeted, and efficient.

Please remember that these are not plans you will have to follow for life. They will get you where you need to be, and then you can move on to the maintenance phase in Part 2. Also, my community is always there to provide even more support, delicious recipes, and motivation to help you stay there. My ultimate goal is to create a community so savvy in nutrition that each person's success, glowing health, and on-fire metabolism will inspire and help others. The best teachers in the world are no longer needed by their students. That's when love replaces need.

Because my weight loss methods are nutrient-driven, you will need to eat in a particular way and style, with targeted foods at different times of the day and throughout the week. There will be purposeful rhythm to your eating, based on the current condition of your metabolism. You will ingest those foods that contain the micronutrients and enzymes you need for fat burning. You will digest those foods fully, completely breaking them down to free up micronutrients and enzymes that convert stored fat to a usable form. Finally, you will absorb those micronutrients and convert fat into fuel for energy (rather than just breaking down the fat on your belly and redepositing it on your butt).

This is the process, but depending on the state of your metabolism, you will require different micronutrient combinations and timing, to customize fat burning and weight loss to your current condition. That's what we're going to find out right now.

The reason I personalize your MIS rather than giving one plan for everyone is that I know the best way to make sure my clients are *not* successful is to treat them like the person who came in before them, or the person who is coming in after them, rather than treating them like the person they are, sitting right in front of me at that moment in time. Your MIS determines how much and what kind of food is right for you over the next fourteen days.

Once we calculate the score, we will carry it throughout the rest of this chapter so you can understand exactly what's coming. Grab your pencil and get ready to create a personalized plan to get up to 14 pounds off fast, while remaking your metabolism for keeping it off or preparing you to keep going to lose even more fat.

CALCULATING YOUR MIS SCORE

To calculate your MIS, divide 14 pounds, which is your maximum weight loss goal for the next fourteen days, by your current body weight in pounds, taken first thing in the morning. Multiply that number by 100 to get your MIS, like this:

Metabolic Intervention Score

(14 pounds ÷ current body weight, taken first thing
in the morning) x 100 = MIS

14 pounds ÷ [_____] x 100 =

current body weight, taken first thing in the morning

[_____]

MIS

PERSONALIZED MEAL MAP:

Meal Map A: If your MIS is 10 or greater.
Meal Map B: If your MIS is between 7 and 9.
Meal Map C: If your MIS is 6 or lower.

YOUR MEAL MAP: [_____]

Let's see how this would work with my client Jessica, who had lost a lot of weight, but had been holding steady for a while, getting used to her new 140-pound body. But Jessica is only 5 feet 2 inches tall, and her goal was 130 pounds. When she told me she was ready to get rid of that last 10 pounds, we divided 14 by 140 to get .10, and multiplied that number by 100 to get an MIS of 10. I gave her Meal Map A to use for the next fourteen days.

Another client, Chris, weighed 193 pounds first thing in the morning when he came to me seeking rapid weight loss. He divided 14 pounds by 193 to get .072, and multiplied that number by 100 to get an MIS of 7.2. I gave him Meal Map B to use for the next fourteen days.

Another of my clients, Melissa, once told me she has lost and regained 1,000 pounds over her lifetime. When we calculated her MIS, Melissa's current body weight first thing in the morning was 260. She divided 14 by 260 to get .053, and multiplied that number by 100 to get an MIS of 5.3. I gave her Meal Map C to use for the next fourteen days.

THE RAPID WEIGHT LOSS MEAL MAPS

Your meal map is designed to address your exact level of need for metabolic intervention, so each meal map does this in several different ways, both with different proportions of protein and carbohydrates, and with a different rotational rhythm:

Meal Map A

If you are on Meal Map A, you aren't far from your ideal weight, but those stubborn final pounds want to hang on because your body feels stable where it is. But don't despair—the trick is to focus on higher carbs, especially in the form of fruit, and a little bit less protein. But that doesn't mean you should eat *no protein*. You still need protein to build muscle and structure, but you need it in different amounts and in different ways than someone on another meal map.

If you are doing Meal Map A, your customized plan has:

- More emphasis on carbohydrates, like whole grains, starchy vegetables, and especially fruit, with just enough high-quality protein to build muscle and structure.
- A week divided by four carb-heavier days and three days with more protein.
- Customized portion sizes, which are generally (but not always) a little smaller than for those who have a higher rate of metabolic dysfunction and more weight to lose.

This chart shows you exactly what and how much you will be eating for each meal during parts 1 and 2:

MEAL MAP A

	BREAKFAST	A.M. SNACK	LUNCH	P.M. SNACK	DINNER
PART 1 (Monday–Thursday)	1 SERVING PROTEIN; 1 SERVING VEGETABLES; 1 SERVING FRUIT; 1 SERVING GRAIN-BASED CARBS OR COMPLEX CARBS	1 SERVING FRUIT	1 SERVING PROTEIN; 2 SERVINGS VEGETABLES; 1 SERVING FRUIT	1 SERVING FRUIT	1 SERVING PROTEIN; 1 SERVING VEGETABLES; 1 SERVING COMPLEX CARBS (NOT GRAIN-BASED)
PART 2 (Friday–Sunday)	1 SERVING PROTEIN; 1 SERVING VEGETABLES; 1 SERVING FRUIT	1 SERVING FRUIT; 1 SERVING HEALTHY FAT	1 SERVING PROTEIN; 1 SERVING VEGETABLES; 1 SERVING HEALTHY FAT	1 SERVING FRUIT; 1 SERVING HEALTHY FAT	1 SERVING PROTEIN; 1 SERVING VEGETABLES; 1 SERVING HEALTHY FAT

A blank version of your meal map, which you will fill out with the foods or recipes you choose to eat each day according to the food categories and portions in the above chart, along with your daily weight, water intake, and exercise choices, will look like this:

MEAL MAP A

	A.M. WEIGHT	BREAKFAST	A.M. SNACK	LUNCH	P.M. SNACK	DINNER	OZ. OF WATER PER DAY	EXERCISE
PART 1 MONDAY								
TUESDAY								
WEDNESDAY								
THURSDAY								
PART 2 FRIDAY								
SATURDAY								
SUNDAY								

Meal Map B

If you are doing Meal Map B, your customized plan has:

- A balance of protein and carbs, to help you lose and then stabilize your easily shifting weight.
- A week divided by three carb-heavier days and four low-carb, higher-protein days.
- Customized portion sizes, in a moderate range between what you would have in Meal Maps C or A.

This chart shows you exactly what and how much you will be eating for each meal during parts 1 and 2:

MEAL MAP B

	BREAKFAST	A.M. SNACK	LUNCH	P.M. SNACK	DINNER
PART 1 (Monday–Wednesday)	1 SERVING PROTEIN 2 SERVINGS VEGETABLES 1 SERVING FRUIT 1 SERVING GRAIN-BASED CARBS OR COMPLEX CARBS	1 SERVING FRUIT	1 SERVING PROTEIN 2 SERVINGS VEGETABLES	1 SERVING FRUIT	1 SERVING PROTEIN 2 SERVINGS VEGETABLES 1 SERVING COMPLEX CARBS (NOT GRAIN-BASED)
PART 2 (Thursday–Sunday)	2 SERVINGS PROTEIN 1 SERVING VEGETABLES 1 SERVING HEALTHY FAT	1 SERVING PROTEIN 1 SERVING HEALTHY FAT	1 SERVING PROTEIN 2 SERVINGS VEGETABLES 1 SERVING HEALTHY FAT	1 SERVING PROTEIN 1 SERVING HEALTHY FAT	1 SERVING PROTEIN 2 SERVINGS VEGETABLES 1 SERVING HEALTHY FAT

A blank version of your meal map, which you will fill out with the foods or recipes you choose to eat each day according to the food categories and portions in the above chart, along with your daily weight, water intake, and exercise choices, will look like this:

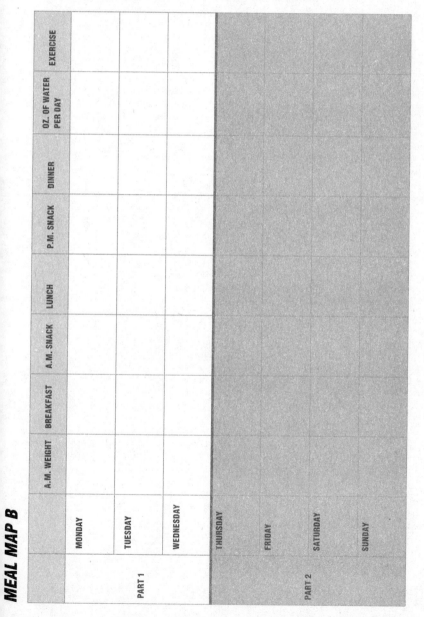

MEAL MAP B

	A.M. WEIGHT	BREAKFAST	A.M. SNACK	LUNCH	P.M. SNACK	DINNER	OZ. OF WATER PER DAY	EXERCISE
MONDAY								
TUESDAY								
WEDNESDAY								
THURSDAY								
FRIDAY								
SATURDAY								
SUNDAY								

PART 1

PART 2

Meal Map C

If you are doing Meal Map C, your customized plan has:

- A focus on protein. Of all the plans, you will be consuming the most protein. You still need carbs for their unique micronutrients, fiber, and energy. They nourish your adrenals, help to calm the stress response, and provide easily accessible energy, but for Meal Map C, carbs play a supporting role to protein.
- A week divided by three carb-heavier days and four low-carb, higher-protein days.
- Customized portion sizes. Because your metabolism needs the most intervention, your portion sizes are the largest. Food is your catalyst for change.

This chart shows you exactly what and how much you will be eating for each meal during parts 1 and 2:

MEAL MAP C

	BREAKFAST	A.M. SNACK	LUNCH	P.M. SNACK	DINNER
PART 1 (Monday–Wednesday)	2 SERVINGS PROTEIN 2 SERVINGS VEGETABLES 1 SERVING FRUIT 1 SERVING GRAIN-BASED CARB OR COMPLEX CARB	1 SERVING FRUIT	1 SERVING PROTEIN 2 SERVINGS VEGETABLES 2 SERVINGS FAT	2 SERVINGS FRUIT	2 SERVINGS PROTEIN 2 SERVINGS VEGETABLES 1 SERVING COMPLEX CARBOHYDRATES (NOT GRAIN-BASED)
PART 2 (Thursday–Sunday)	2 SERVINGS PROTEIN 2 SERVINGS VEGETABLES 1 SERVING HEALTHY FAT	1 SERVING PROTEIN 1 SERVING HEALTHY FAT	1 SERVING PROTEIN 2 SERVINGS VEGETABLES 2 SERVINGS HEALTHY FAT	1 SERVING PROTEIN 1 SERVING HEALTHY FAT	1 SERVING PROTEIN 2 SERVINGS VEGETABLES 2 SERVINGS HEALTHY FAT

A blank version of your meal map, which you will fill out with the foods or recipes you choose to eat each day according to the food categories and portions in the above chart, along with your daily weight, water intake, and exercise choices, will look like this:

MEAL MAP C

	A.M. WEIGHT	BREAKFAST	A.M. SNACK	LUNCH	P.M. SNACK	DINNER	OZ. OF WATER PER DAY	EXERCISE
MONDAY								
TUESDAY								
WEDNESDAY								
THURSDAY								
FRIDAY								
SATURDAY								
SUNDAY								

PART 1

PART 2

THE METABOLISM REVOLUTION FOOD LIST

This list contains only those foods that I know from my clinical experience and education to be particularly good at burning fat rapidly. I don't want you to deviate from this food list while doing the Metabolism Revolution, but you can deviate *within the list*, substituting any item in a particular group (like protein, complex carb, fruit, or vegetable) for any other in the recipes on pages 123 to 193.

METABOLISM REVOLUTION FOOD LIST

FREE FOODS (UNLIMITED)

These can be incorporated into any meal at any time in unlimited quantities.

100% monk fruit/lo han	Lemons
100% pure stevia	Limes
Birch xylitol	Mustard, pure (no additives)
Celery	Onions
Dried or fresh herbs and spices	Pepper: black, red, red pepper flakes
Egg whites	Raw cacao
Garlic	Sea salt
Ginger	Vinegar, pure (no additives)
Horseradish	

FRUITS: 1 CUP = 1 PORTION

These may be fresh or frozen and may be served in combination.

Apples	Peaches
Berries, all	Pears
Cherries	Pineapple
Grapefruit	Plums
Mangoes	
Melons, all	
Nectarines	
Oranges	

VEGETABLES: 2 CUPS RAW / 1 CUP COOKED = 1 PORTION

These may be fresh or frozen, served raw or cooked, and can be served in combination.

Asparagus

Beets, all

Broccoli/Broccolini

Cabbage

Carrots

Cauliflower

Cucumbers

Green beans, yellow beans, wax beans

Leafy greens and lettuces

Mushrooms, all

Onions, all

Peppers, all

Radishes

Squashes, all

NON-GRAIN-BASED COMPLEX CARBS: ½ CUP COOKED = 1 PORTION

Beans/legumes (except peanuts, green peas, and soy)

Quinoa

Sweet potatoes/yams

Wild rice

GRAINS: ½ CUP COOKED = 1 PORTION

Brown rice

Buckwheat

Kamut

Oats

Spelt

PROTEINS: 4 OUNCES (OR 2 EGGS) = 1 PORTION

Organic, free-range, and antibiotic-free is preferred. Select nitrite-free, with no additives, sugars, or preservatives.

Beef

Buffalo

Chicken

Eggs, whole

Fish, wild-caught

Lamb

Pork

Shrimp

Turkey

Wild game

VEGETABLE PROTEINS

Legumes (such as lentils, black beans, white beans, refried beans, etc.—*no peanuts*), ¾ cup

Mushrooms, any type, 3 cups raw

Tempeh, 4 ounces raw (the only allowed soy product)

HEALTHY FAT

These can be served in combination.

Avocado, ¼

Hummus, ¼ cup

Nut and seed butters, from raw nuts and
seeds only, 2 tablespoons

Nuts and seeds, raw only, ¼ cup

Oils (avocado, coconut, grapeseed,
olive, safflower, sunflower, walnut oil),
2 tablespoons

Olives, 8 to 10 olives

Raw coconut meat, ¼ cup

Safflower mayonnaise, 2 tablespoons

Mix and Match

As you begin this plan, you may notice that the amount of protein and vegetables in your plan is pretty large, especially for Meal Map C, where protein is crucial for metabolic repair and vegetables are important for providing enzymes to digest all that protein. But I get that it can feel like too much. When your meal map lists two servings of protein or vegetables at a meal, you don't have to eat two servings of the same thing. You can mix and match, choosing two different proteins and/or two different vegetables. For example, you can have 2 eggs and turkey sausage instead of 4 eggs, or 4 ounces chicken breast and ¾ cup black beans instead of 8 ounces chicken breast. With vegetables, you can get even more creative. If your meal map says 4 cups vegetables, you can choose 2 cups each of two kinds, or 1 cup each of four different vegetables. The more variety, the more micronutrients.

The Elephant in the Room

You might have already noticed that my list contains no wheat, no dairy, no sugar, no soy (except tempeh), no corn, and no alcohol. I have selected the foods on this food list to zero in on weight loss, and any additions will dilute the effect and slow down your progress. I'll say more about additional foods in the second half of this book, especially in chapter 9, which is all about metabolic disruptors. For now, just know that for the next fourteen days, your choices are limited for a good reason. I want you to focus on what you are doing, not what you *aren't* doing. That is the mind-set that will lead to success.

But now I'm going to address the elephant in the room. I'm going to talk about coffee. And not just coffee, but caffeine in general. I'm going to talk about coffee because many people's knee-jerk reaction is "No coffee? No way!" Hear me out.

American runs on coffee, or so they say. Some of you may run on a cup of strong black tea, or even a cola, to get you through the morning or that afternoon slump. But it's important for you to know that caffeine is a potent adrenal gland stressor. Your adrenal glands are instrumental in keeping your stress hormones under control and also in regulating your blood sugar. Rapid weight loss is much more difficult with stress hormones like cortisol pumping through your system, and it is nearly impossible when you are having big blood sugar spikes followed by surges of insulin. Your body is designed to provide you with the energy you need to get through your day without stimulants. When you give it the nutrients it needs for energy metabolism instead of "fake" energy from caffeine, your energy will be steadier, last longer, and feel better, with no jitters, shaky hands, or nervousness, and no afternoon crashes, either.

A lot of people try to argue with me by defending coffee and other caffeinated beverages. They say things like "But coffee kills my appetite so I eat less" or "But coffee helps makes me sharper and smarter." Coffee is an appetite suppressant only for low-carb, low-calorie dieters, and that is the kind of diet I do not condone, because if you ever go off it, you will be prone to rapid weight gain. And as for sharper thinking, that comes from flooding your brain with micronutrients it needs to grow more neurons, and from regular exercise, which washes your brain with brain-derived neurotrophic factor (BDNF), a protein that nurtures and stimulates your brain cells. Coffee has nothing to do with it.

I would love nothing more than for you to tell me, "Haylie, I finally quit coffee, and I've never felt better or more energetic in my life." You would not be the first person to tell me that, and you won't be the last, but I hope you *will* join the growing legion of people who have freed themselves from the tyranny of caffeine. And after just three or four days, when the headache clears (which is the proof of your addiction), you'll see the light. And you won't regret it.

YOUR MEAL MAP EXERCISE PLAN

Each meal map also comes with an exercise plan customized to best take advantage of the meal map's particular protein-carb balance, as well as your particular need for metabolic repair. Your meal map will specify how much cardio to do and whether or not weight lifting is beneficial for you right now, and will also have specific guidance for Metabolic Intervention Exercises (MIEs). Here are some *guidelines for cardio, weight lifting, and MIE—options, frequency, and intensity.*

Cardio Guidelines

Cardio doesn't just burn fat. It also releases endorphins and catecholamines that make you feel calm and good, so your body can stop panicking and hoarding stored fat. Choose any activity from this list for your cardio:

- Biking—outdoors, on a stationary bike, or in a Spin class
- Boxing/kickboxing
- Brisk/power walking outdoors, on a track, or on a treadmill
- Dancing or dance classes like Zumba
- Elliptical trainer

- Hiking
- Rowing, in an actual boat or on a machine
- Running/jogging outdoors, on a track, or on a treadmill
- Sports with sustained activity like volleyball and basketball
- Stair climbing, on any set of actual stairs or on a stair-climbing machine
- Step aerobics class
- Swimming
- Yoga that keeps you moving, like hot yoga or Vinyasa yoga

Your goal is to raise your heart rate to between 120 and 140 beats per minute for 20 to 35 minutes, but not to go over 145 beats per minute. The level of intensity will depend on your level of fitness. For some of my clients, climbing a short flight of stairs will raise their heart rate that much. For others, it takes running a 6-minute mile to get their heart rates up high enough. You can track your heart rate on most newer fitness watches, or with a heart rate monitor strap around your chest or wrist. Some workout equipment also tracks your heart rate for you if you hold your finger over the sensor while exercising.

While cardio is important, please observe the upper limit as well. When you are using food for weight loss and strategically stimulating muscle development, preserving and building muscle is crucial for success. When your heart rate elevates too high and exercise becomes strenuous, muscle mass can be broken down. Your current muscle mass is sacred to us over the next fourteen days. It is going to help you achieve rapid weight loss, so you cannot afford to lose any muscle during this time. If you are in the habit of strenuous cardio, you will be able to get back to it, but right now, keep your heart rate under 145 bpm, so you aren't undermining your efforts to repair your metabolism.

Weight-Lifting Exercise Guidelines

If you are using Meal Maps B or C, you will also be lifting weights once or twice every week. Choose a different day to lift weights than the day you do cardio. Use free weights, weight machines, resistance bands or balls, or your own body weight to work these muscles. To stimulate aggressive fat burn, work with stacked reps in sets of 3. Start with 8 reps, then 6 reps, then 4 reps. The weight should be heavy enough that you can just complete the reps to muscle exhaustion. If you can do a lot more reps, then you need to increase your weight. Always keep your body in a stable, supported position to avoid injury, and if you have an injury already (like a rotator cuff tear or knee ligament tear), don't stress that area with weights. Focus on other areas instead. You will still get the benefits. For our purposes over the next fourteen days, the best way to use weights to your advantage is to focus on your choice of any three large muscle groups on any given weight day. On subsequent days, change the muscle groups, rotating through the following list:

- Quadriceps and hamstrings (your thigh muscles)
- Gluteus (your butt muscles)
- Soleus (your calf muscles)
- Pectorals (your chest muscles)
- Abdominals (your stomach muscles)
- Trapezius and latissimus dorsa (your back muscles)
- Deltoids (your shoulder muscles)
- Biceps and triceps (your upper arm muscles)

If you aren't sure what exercises to do for your chosen muscle group, ask a trainer at your gym for help, or check out the exercises on hayliepomroy.com organized by weight group. You can also look up exercises for each of these muscle groups in books or on fitness websites.

Metabolic Intervention Exercises (MIEs)

MIEs are supported or passive activities like massage, infrared sauna, and Epsom salt baths that are critical for rapid weight loss success.

You will be making changes to your diet and exercise routine, and the calming, stress-reversing action of MIEs will minimize stress hormone production so your body can more easily get into fat-burning mode. Remember that when your body experiences chronic stress, it hoards fat. MIEs reverse that response. MIEs also stimulate your circulation, increase blood flow and lymphatic flow, and facilitate waste removal. On top of all that, they feel great, so don't skip them.

Somebody has to take out the trash, and these exercises are superheroes in that department. Don't underestimate them.

If you can, do these exercises on days when you are not doing any other exercises. Here are my favorite MIEs:

- Massage
- Dry skin brushing
- Epsom salt baths
- Infrared sauna
- Physical therapy
- Acupuncture
- Gentle yoga or simple stretching

MIEs are also an excellent option for those who have mobility issues. If you cannot do regular cardio and/or weight lifting, you could incorporate an MIE four or five times per week instead of traditional exercise. I talk more about this in the FAQs in chapter 5.

Here are your customized exercise prescriptions, per meal map.

Meal Map A

Cardio is your friend. You don't need the aggressive historical fat scavenging actions of weight lifting over the next fourteen days. Rather than build structure right now, you want to focus on getting rid of those stubborn remaining pounds that haven't responded to your previous efforts. When someone doesn't have a large amount of body fat mass to lose, there is typically less visceral fat, and the fat you want to get rid of is more integrated into your muscles and fascia. When that happens, we need to focus on a lot of vasodilation and increased blood flow, which is what cardio accomplishes for you. But don't sweat it—if you love lifting weights, you can go back to it. Just take a break for these fourteen days.

- *Cardio:* 3 or 4 times per week, to raise your heart rate to between 120 and 140 beats per minute for 20 to 35 minutes for each session.
- *Weights:* No weight lifting during the 14-day program.
- *Metabolic Intervention Exercises:* Minimum of 1 time per week.

Meal Map B

You fall right in between the weight-training-centric needs of those on Meal Map C and the cardio requirements of those on Meal Map A. You need a balanced combination of both the stress-relieving, fat-burning, vasodilating effects of cardio, and the potent fat-releasing and muscle-building effects of weight training—the best of both worlds.

- *Cardio:* 2 or 3 times per week, to raise your heart rate to between 120 and 140 beats per minute for 20 to 35 minutes for each session.
- *Weights:* 1 time per week, focusing on 3 major muscle groups for each session.
- *Metabolic Intervention Exercises:* Minimum of 1 time per week.

Meal Map C

If you are using Meal Map C, weights are your friend. You will be doing some cardio because cardio dilates your blood vessels for more efficient circulation and also reduces the stress response, but weight lifting is critical for people experiencing weight loss resistance who have accumulated a significant amount of visceral fat. Weight lifting causes microtears to the muscle, which prompts your body to excrete an enzyme called creatine kinase. This enzyme scavenges the resistant outer "shell" around visceral fat so it can be more easily released into the bloodstream. This is a powerful way to break up and release fat stores you may have been holding on to for decades.

- *Cardio:* 2 or 3 times per week, to raise your heart rate to between 120 and 140 beats per minute for 20 to 35 minutes for each session.
- *Weights:* 2 times per week, focusing on 3 major muscle groups for each session.
- *Metabolic Intervention Exercises:* Minimum of 2 times per week.

THE RAPID WEIGHT LOSS RULES

No matter what meal map you are following, these are general healthy guidelines to follow that are conducive to rapid weight loss in any situation. I recommend practicing these habits even when you aren't working to lose weight quickly. They are rules 4 life that will always benefit your efforts at both weight loss and weight maintenance. For the next fourteen days, while you are on the Metabolism Revolution program, they are nonnegotiable. Here are the rules:

Eat 35 Times Per Week

Eat five times per day (a total of thirty-five meals and snacks per week). To stoke your metabolic fire and burn away fat at the rapid pace we are going for during the next fourteen days, it is essential to eat often. You must keep kindling that fire. Do not skip any meals or snacks.

Eat Within 30 Minutes of Waking

Eat within 30 minutes of waking. This is no time to skip breakfast, or you douse the fire at the beginning of your day. Even if you must swap a snack with breakfast in order to get out the door in time, eat something right away. After 30 minutes, you have already depressed your metabolic fire and you will have a harder time getting it going again.

Eat Every 2 to 4 Hours

Eat every 2 to 4 hours (except, obviously, when you are sleeping). In some of my other books, I say not to go longer than 3 to 4 hours, but eating every 2 hours is just fine and a good way to keep your metabolism burning. *Never* go longer than 4 hours without a meal or snack when you are awake, or your metabolic fire will begin to die down. This is extremely important.

Make the 14-Day Commitment

Stay on the plan for fourteen days. If you see big results after one week, don't get satisfied and quit. You need to do the entire fourteen days for the weight to get off and stay off. When you lose weight quickly at the beginning, you need to solidify those results. If your weight is stubborn, you may also find that you lose most of it in the second half. No matter what your Metabolic Intervention Score is today, you need fourteen solid days of repair to get the job done, and get it done right.

Stick to Your Split

Your assigned meal map has a 4/3 or 3/4 split, with one style of eating for the first part of the week, and a different style of eating for the second half. This split is specifically for the purpose of fueling rapid weight loss, so don't stray from it.

Drink Half Your Body Weight in Ounces of Water Every Day

When you lose weight quickly, your body is shedding fat, fluid, and the waste products of metabolism. Help that process along and stay hydrated by getting in the habit of drinking half your body weight in ounces of clean spring water per day. For example, if you weigh 180 pounds, you would drink 90 ounces of water every day. I like to fill up a jug with my water for the day and pour glasses from that until it's gone so I don't have to keep track of my ounces, but whatever way works for you is great.

Eat Organic Whenever Possible

I understand that organic food isn't always available or affordable, so I don't absolutely require it. However, whenever you can, keep the pesticides and pharmaceuticals out of your food by eating organic, *especially* when it comes to meat, and vegetables and fruits that you eat without peeling. These agricultural chemicals are metabolic disruptors (see chapter 9). When your liver must focus on processing toxins (not just food chemicals but also environmental pollution, alcohol, and pharmaceuticals), it can't focus on processing fat. Organic food and a clean environment make your liver's job easier, and weight loss faster.

Don't Eat Off-Plan

The foods I've chosen for you are specifically designed to get the weight off fast, so stick to your food list. If you are tempted to ask me, "But, Haylie, can I have X, Y, or Z?," just assume the answer is "Not for the next fourteen days." You can, however, swap like items with other items on the list—fruit for fruit, vegetable for vegetable, protein for protein, etc. For instance, if you don't like asparagus but you love cucumber, you can swap those in equal portions. But don't swap for something that isn't on the list, like tomatoes or jicama. Those are off the list for the next fourteen days for good reason, even though they are on some of the food lists in some of my other plans. Each plan has specific goals, so don't eat off-plan.

Choose Your 14 Days Wisely

Before you jump into the plan, you'll need to pull out your calendar and find a fourteen-day period where you don't have a lot of super-stressful things going on. Don't do it when you are moving, or sending your last child off to college, or starting a new job. Don't do it when you are going to be on vacation, or you have a lot of high-intensity work stuff happening.

But don't put it off, either. Life is full of stressful times, and you can't ever avoid them completely. Just do your best to find a fourteen-day period when you can exercise control over what you eat and when you exercise. That's the most important thing. It's not that you can't do the Metabolism Revolution when you are traveling or going to a restaurant. In fact, in the next chapter, I'll show you how my client Cathy managed to eat out a few times during her fourteen-day plan, and also how my client Jeanine was able to take her whole family out to eat for their traditional Friday-night family dinner. But it's easier to do it when you make your food at home, so I encourage you to do that most of the time over the next fourteen days. Choosing a fourteen-day period when this is at least mostly possible will help everything sail along with less effort.

Choose a Start Date

Also consider your starting day carefully. Many of my clients like to start on a Monday, just because it makes sense to them to start at the beginning of the week. Then you will end on a Sunday, and in two weeks from this Monday, you'll feel like a whole new you. But starting on a Monday isn't required. You can start on any day of the week. Planning is everything.

Now let's take a look at the process that will propel you straight through those fourteen days so you come out the other side feeling like you've experienced a Metabolism Revolution.

4

YOUR METABOLISM REVOLUTION
WEIGHT LOSS PLAN

Now that you have all the information you need—your ideal weight, your degree of metabolic dysfunction, your Metabolic Intervention Score, your meal map assignment, and the philosophies behind the meal maps and exercise plans for each meal map—it's time to get excited, because the next two weeks will be filled with delicious food, enjoyable movement, and dramatic metabolic transformation.

In this chapter, find your blank meal map (A, B, or C) for planning your fourteen days. It tells you everything you need to do. You can map it all out before you start, or go day by day, recording what you do as you go along. Some of my clients like to get super-organized with all the food purchased, precooked, and frozen into portions before they begin. Others like to shop every day and cook as they go along. It depends on your time, schedule, and personal inclinations.

You can also choose foods that work for each category (protein, vegetable, fruit, complex carb, etc.), piecing your meals together like a puzzle, or you can choose recipes from chapter 6, which automatically comply with your needs when you prepare them according to your meal map. You can make a different recipe every night, or choose the ones that intrigue you and cook big batches before you start, freezing your portions individually to save time. (For those who want to cook even less, check out my Super-Simple Supported Plan on page 303.) I've had clients choose and prep their food in many different ways. It's purely a matter of personal preference.

I've had many clients go successfully through this plan, so before I give you your detailed meal map to fill out for the next two weeks, let's meet some people who have been there and done that: Sue, Cathy, and Jeanine. Sue's Metabolic Intervention Score resulted in a match for Meal Map A, Cathy got Meal Map B, and Jeanine got Meal Map C. Let's take a closer look at how each of them navigated their fourteen days.

MEET SUE AND HER MEAL MAP A

Sue is a twentysomething client of mine with a high-profile job, a supportive boyfriend, and a cute apartment in a large city. She came to me weighing 135 pounds, and although for some people this would be a dream weight, for Sue, it was a plateau. For her slight frame, 128 pounds was the perfect weight for her—the weight at which she knew she felt her best. But she hadn't been able to get there. She had been stuck in the 130s, going up and down, for five years, and just couldn't seem to break through that barrier. She told me she didn't need to lose 14 pounds in fourteen days. She would be overjoyed just to lose those stubborn 7 pounds that stood between her and her best body. Could I help?

Of course. We sat down together and did the calculations, and her Metabolic Intervention Score coincided with Meal Map A, so that is what we chose for her. We also calculated her water intake. Remember, I want you to drink half your body weight in ounces of water every day during the fourteen-day plan. For Sue, who weighed 135 pounds, that meant (rounding up) she needed to drink 68 ounces of water per day. Since half a gallon is 64 ounces, I suggested that she drink 4 ounces first thing in the morning, then fill a half-gallon pitcher with water and keep it in the refrigerator. She filled her water bottle from that pitcher throughout the day so she didn't have to keep track of her ounces. As she lost weight, her water intake would go down accordingly. Although Sue wasn't a big fan of water, a few slices of fresh lemon and lime in the pitcher helped her get it down, and once she was into the habit, she began to crave it.

For exercise, we looked at the Meal Map A exercise plan, and Sue saw that she needed to do three or four sessions of cardio each week along with a minimum of one Metabolic Intervention Exercise (MIE). Sue loves to take step classes at her local gym or work out on the elliptical trainer, so she scheduled these in, along with a massage during the first week and a session in her gym's infrared sauna on the second week.

The next thing we did was look at the recipes (chapter 6). We flipped through them all, and she picked out the ones she thought looked good and that used foods she knew she liked. She also picked a few things she'd never tried before, like Savory Oats, because she thought they sounded interesting and wanted to expand her palate (and micronutrient intake). I gave her a blank meal map and she filled out the meals she wanted to have. Then we made a shopping list of ingredients from the recipes. We found the Meal Map A column in each recipe and wrote down what she would need, multiplying each recipe by the number of times she planned to have it during the fourteen days. Before she started, she cooked most of the meals in batches and froze individual portions. Then she followed her meal map through the fourteen days. Every night, she looked ahead to see what she would be eating the next day and took those meals out of the freezer. She told me she hardly spent any time in the kitchen once the fourteen days started, which made it easier for her to focus on getting all her meals, snacks, exercises, and water in each day.

Sue broke through her plateau on Day 10, and landed solidly on her goal weight by Day 14. She was so proud of herself, and I was proud of her, too. Now she is holding steady on the Fast Metabolism 4 Life plan from the second half of this book. Here is her completed meal map. Take a close look to see everything she did to comply with Meal Map A.

MEAL MAP A: SUE (Recipes start on page 123.)

Week One

		A.M. WEIGHT	BREAKFAST	A.M. SNACK	LUNCH	P.M. SNACK	DINNER	OZ. OF WATER PER DAY	EXERCISE
PART 1	MONDAY	135	SAVORY OATS WITH APPLE SLICES	ASIAN PEAR	BROILED COD WITH NECTARINE SALSA OVER MIXED GREENS	CHERRIES	STEAK, MUSHROOM, AND SWEET POTATO KEBABS	68 OUNCES	STEP CLASS
	TUESDAY	134.2	BREAKFAST HASH	STRAWBERRIES	ONE-PAN TROPICAL CHICKEN	ORANGE	LEMON-BASIL PORK CHOPS WITH WILD RICE	67 OUNCES	REST
	WEDNESDAY	133.7	SAVORY OATS WITH APPLE SLICES	ASIAN PEAR	BROILED COD WITH NECTARINE SALSA OVER MIXED GREENS	CHERRIES	STEAK, MUSHROOM, AND SWEET POTATO KEBABS	67 OUNCES	ELLIPTICAL TRAINER
	THURSDAY	133.1	BREAKFAST HASH	STRAWBERRIES	ONE-PAN TROPICAL CHICKEN	ORANGE	LEMON-BASIL PORK CHOPS WITH WILD RICE	67 OUNCES	STEP CLASS
PART 2	FRIDAY	132.4	STUFFED PEPPER BREAKFAST WITH PEACHES	APPLE WITH ALMOND BUTTER	SHRIMP SALAD	PINEAPPLE CHUNKS WITH SHREDDED COCONUT	PISTACHIO PORK WITH BROCCOLI	66 OUNCES	MASSAGE
	SATURDAY	131.9	SCRAMBLED SALMON CUPS	PINEAPPLE CHUNKS WITH SHREDDED COCONUT	TUNA-STUFFED AVOCADO	APPLE WITH ALMOND BUTTER	RAINBOW CHICKEN AND VEGETABLES	66 OUNCES	REST
	SUNDAY	131.1	STUFFED PEPPER BREAKFAST AND MIXED BERRIES	APPLE WITH ALMOND BUTTER	SHRIMP SALAD	PINEAPPLE CHUNKS WITH SHREDDED COCONUT	PISTACHIO PORK WITH BROCCOLI	66 OUNCES	ELLIPTICAL TRAINER

Week Two

	A.M. WEIGHT	BREAKFAST	A.M. SNACK	LUNCH	P.M. SNACK	DINNER	OZ. OF WATER PER DAY	EXERCISE
PART 1								
MONDAY	130.5	BLACK BEAN SCRAMBLE WITH MELON	KIWI	CHICKEN BACON FRUIT SALAD	BLUEBERRIES	STEAK AND QUINOA BOWL	65 OUNCES	STEP CLASS
TUESDAY	130	SAVORY OATS WITH APPLE SLICES	RASPBERRIES	PINEAPPLE-CUCUMBER SALAD WITH SEA BASS	ASIAN PEAR	CAJUN SHRIMP AND BLACK BEANS	65 OUNCES	REST
WEDNESDAY	129.6	BLACK BEAN SCRAMBLE WITH MELON	KIWI	CHICKEN BACON FRUIT SALAD	BLUEBERRIES	STEAK AND QUINOA BOWL	65 OUNCES	ELLIPTICAL TRAINER
THURSDAY	129.1	SAVORY OATS WITH APPLE SLICES	RASPBERRIES	PINEAPPLE-CUCUMBER SALAD WITH SEA BASS	ASIAN PEAR	CAJUN SHRIMP AND BLACK BEANS	65 OUNCES	STEP CLASS
PART 2								
FRIDAY	128.7	SCRAMBLED SALMON CUPS	MANGO CHUNKS WITH SHREDDED COCONUT	LEMON SHRIMP BOWL	APPLE WITH ALMOND BUTTER	GRILLED STEAK WITH AVOCADO SALSA	64 OUNCES	INFRARED SAUNA
SATURDAY	128.3	STUFFED PEPPER BREAKFAST WITH PEACHES	APPLE WITH ALMOND BUTTER	TUNA-STUFFED AVOCADO	MANGO CHUNKS WITH SHREDDED COCONUT	RAINBOW CHICKEN AND VEGETABLES	64 OUNCES	REST
SUNDAY	128	SCRAMBLED SALMON CUPS	MANGO CHUNKS WITH SHREDDED COCONUT	LEMON SHRIMP BOWL	APPLE WITH ALMOND BUTTER	GRILLED STEAK WITH AVOCADO SALSA	64 OUNCES	ELLIPTICAL TRAINER

otice how Sue didn't make something new every single day. She cooked some things ahead in batches before she started and froze them in portions. Instead of fourteen different breakfasts, Sue enjoyed a total of five breakfasts—three different recipes for Part 1 and two different recipes for Part 2. She made four lunches for Part 1 and three for Part 2. She also made a total of four dinners for Part 1 and three dinners for Part 2. This greatly reduced the time she spent cooking, and was more cost-effective than buying ingredients for forty-two different meals and twenty-eight different snacks.

For example, Sue had Savory Oats for breakfast four times over the course of fourteen days, but she only made this recipe once. She quadrupled the recipe, then divided the oats into four separate portions and froze them. The night before she planned to eat Savory Oats for breakfast, she removed one portion from the freezer. In the morning, all she had to do was heat it up and add some fresh fruit. Or she could have even put her frozen berries in there when she heated it up. Or when she packed it up. You can do it any way you want, with as much pre-prep and as much fresh prep at you want.

If you are using Meal Map A, this is your blank form. You can imitate Sue, or do your own thing. You can use this blank Meal Map A to plan your whole week ahead, so you know exactly what you will be having and how many portions to prepare from any recipe you use. Or if you like to cook as you go, use this to keep track of everything you eat and do, either using recipes or just choosing foods from the list on page 56 based on each day's requirement. Don't forget to track your weight, exercise, and water. Your blank meal map is the place to keep track of everything so you stay organized. A reminder of your exercise plan is located after your blank meal map. (If you are doing Meal Map B or C, use the form on page 88 or 100, respectively.)

Meal Map A (Metabolic Intervention Score 10 or greater)

Week One—Part 1

	A.M. WEIGHT	BREAKFAST	A.M. SNACK	LUNCH	P.M. SNACK	DINNER	OZ. OF WATER PER DAY	EXERCISE
MONDAY		RECIPE: OR 1 P: 1 V: 1 F: 1 G OR CC:	1 F:	RECIPE: OR 1 P: 2 V: 1 F:	1 F:	RECIPE: OR 1 P: 1 V: 1 CC:		
TUESDAY		RECIPE: OR 1 P: 1 V: 1 F: 1 G OR CC:	1 F:	RECIPE: OR 1 P: 2 V: 1 F:	1 F:	RECIPE: OR 1 P: 1 V: 1 CC:		
WEDNESDAY		RECIPE: OR 1 P: 1 V: 1 F: 1 G OR CC:	1 F:	RECIPE: OR 1 P: 2 V: 1 F:	1 F:	RECIPE: OR 1 P: 1 V: 1 CC:		
THURSDAY		RECIPE: OR 1 P: 1 V: 1 F: 1 G OR CC:	1 F:	RECIPE: OR 1 P: 2 V: 1 F:	1 F:	RECIPE: OR 1 P: 1 V: 1 CC:		

PART 1

KEY: P = Protein V = Veggie F = Fruit CC = Complex Carb G = Grain-Based Carb HF = Healthy Fat and Oils

Week One—Part 2

	A.M. WEIGHT	BREAKFAST	A.M. SNACK	LUNCH	P.M. SNACK	DINNER	OZ. OF WATER PER DAY	EXERCISE
FRIDAY		RECIPE: OR 1 P: 1 V: 1 F:	1 F: 1 HF:	RECIPE: OR 1 P: 1 V: 1 HF:	1 P: 1 HF:	RECIPE: OR 1 P: 1 V: 1 HF:		
PART 2 SATURDAY		RECIPE: OR 1 P: 1 V: 1 F:	1 F: 1 HF:	RECIPE: OR 1 P: 1 V: 1 HF:	1 P: 1 HF:	RECIPE: OR 1 P: 1 V: 1 HF:		
SUNDAY		RECIPE: OR 1 P: 1 V: 1 F:	1 F: 1 HF:	RECIPE: OR 1 P: 1 V: 1 HF:	1 P: 1 HF:	RECIPE: OR 1 P: 1 V: 1 HF:		

KEY: P = Protein V = Veggie F = Fruit CC = Complex Carb G = Grain-Based Carb HF = Healthy Fat and Oils

Meal Map A (Metabolic Intervention Score 10 or greater)
Week Two—Part 1

	A.M. WEIGHT	BREAKFAST	A.M. SNACK	LUNCH	P.M. SNACK	DINNER	OZ. OF WATER PER DAY	EXERCISE
MONDAY		RECIPE: OR 1 P: 1 V: 1 F: 1 G OR CC:	1 F:	RECIPE: OR 1 P: 2 V: 1 F:	1 F:	RECIPE: OR 1 P: 1 V: 1 CC:		
TUESDAY		RECIPE: OR 1 P: 1 V: 1 F: 1 G OR CC:	1 F:	RECIPE: OR 1 P: 2 V: 1 F:	1 F:	RECIPE: OR 1 P: 1 V: 1 CC:		
WEDNESDAY		RECIPE: OR 1 P: 1 V: 1 F: 1 G OR CC:	1 F:	RECIPE: OR 1 P: 2 V: 1 F:	1 F:	RECIPE: OR 1 P: 1 V: 1 CC:		
THURSDAY		RECIPE: OR 1 P: 1 V: 1 F: 1 G OR CC:	1 F:	RECIPE: OR 1 P: 2 V: 1 F:	1 F:	RECIPE: OR 1 P: 1 V: 1 CC:		

PART 1

Week Two—Part 2

	A.M. WEIGHT	BREAKFAST	A.M. SNACK	LUNCH	P.M. SNACK	DINNER	OZ. OF WATER PER DAY	EXERCISE
FRIDAY		RECIPE: OR 1 P: 1 V: 1 F:	1 F: 1 HF:	RECIPE: OR 1 P: 1 V: 1 HF:	1 P: 1 HF:	RECIPE: OR 1 P: 1 V: 1 HF:		
PART 2 SATURDAY		RECIPE: OR 1 P: 1 V: 1 F:	1 F: 1 HF:	RECIPE: OR 1 P: 1 V: 1 HF:	1 P: 1 HF:	RECIPE: OR 1 P: 1 V: 1 HF:		
SUNDAY		RECIPE: OR 1 P: 1 V: 1 F:	1 F: 1 HF:	RECIPE: OR 1 P: 1 V: 1 HF:	1 P: 1 HF:	RECIPE: OR 1 P: 1 V: 1 HF:		

KEY: P = Protein V = Veggie F = Fruit CC = Complex Carb G = Grain-Based Carb HF = Healthy Fat and Oils

Meal Map A Recommended Exercise

(See the list of approved cardio and MIE exercises on page 60.)

- *Cardio:* 3 or 4 times per week, to raise your heart rate to between 120 and 140 beats per minute for 20 to 35 minutes for each session.
- *Weights:* No weight lifting during the 14-day program.
- *Metabolic Intervention Exercises:* Minimum of 1 time per week.

MEET CATHY AND HER MEAL MAP B

Cathy is a busy working mom with three young children. She's always running around trying to get everything done and rarely takes any time for herself. She admitted to me that she often eats her kids' leftovers for her meal—some macaroni and cheese, a few green beans, some cookies and milk. In college, she weighed 150 pounds and felt strong and good about herself, but when she came to see me, she had been at 170 pounds since having her third child two years earlier. She said her clothes felt uncomfortable, her stomach was always a little bloated, and she didn't have the energy she felt she needed to be a good mom and also excel at her job. I thought she was a Super Mom, but she didn't feel very super, so we got right to work.

After calculating Cathy's Metabolic Intervention Score, we discovered that she was a match for Meal Map B. Getting down into the 150s in fourteen days sounded great to her. She was inspired and ready, but she warned me that she didn't have much time, and sometimes after work, the whole family went out to dinner because there wasn't time to cook and the kids needed food fast. I explained that many of the meals could be made ahead in portions to feed the whole family. She or her husband would only have to heat them up.

She asked me about business and working lunches, and I told her there were ways to stay on plan in restaurants, too. For example, in Part 1, Meal Map B lunch consists of one serving of protein, two servings of vegetables, and one serving of fruit. I told her to order a big salad with chicken, steak, or salmon and lots of vegetables, hold the cheese and croutons. She could drizzle it with vinegar and have her fruit serving back at the office. Or she could have lettuce wraps with steak or chicken, or sushi rolls with fish and vegetables only (you can ask for sushi rolls without rice), and stay right on plan. I encouraged her to keep a stash of fresh fruit at the office to get in all her required fruit. Part 2 was even easier. For Meal Map B, lunch is one serving of protein, two servings of vegetables, and one serving of healthy fat. She could add olive oil or avocado to her salad or lettuce wraps, or add avocado to her sushi rolls. She felt this was definitely workable for her situation.

Next we looked at her water intake. I told her that since she weighed 170, she would start by drinking 85 ounces of water each day and decrease the water as her weight decreased. Cathy always had a large water bottle with her that held 1 liter, or 33.8 ounces, of water. We figured out that she would need to drink 2½ of these bottles to get in her 85 ounces. She said sometimes she did that anyway, so she would be sure to make that happen every day for the next fourteen days.

According to her Meal Map B suggested exercise, Cathy would need to do cardio two or three times per week, and weight lifting one time per week, plus a minimum of one MIE. Cathy said she was a bath person, often relaxing in a hot bath after the kids went to bed. She decided to buy some lavender-scented Epsom salts and use that as her MIE, since she didn't think she would have time to go get a massage, physical therapy, or acupuncture. She loved to jog but hadn't done it in a while, so she chose jogging as her cardio. Her husband had a set of weights in the basement. She said she would dust them off and find one day each week to target some major muscle groups.

Finally, we went through all the recipes in chapter 6. She circled the ones that included foods her whole family liked, and we worked them into her blank meal map. She counted up five portions for every time she made each recipe and made her grocery list based on this. It was less expensive than she expected because she could buy meat and frozen vegetables in larger packages for lower prices. We looked at her calendar and scheduled a weekend for cooking. She made all the meals ahead of time, dividing everything into large zip-top bags that held five portions each (for some meals she knew would be especially popular, like the Sausage and Roasted Veggies and the Chicken Black Bean Tacos, she made eight servings to allow her husband and kids to have second helpings). Everything went into the freezer, and then she was ready. She was excited and motivated because the plan felt doable and not intimidating.

She kicked off her plan on a Monday, and two weeks later, she was down to 158 pounds, for a total loss of 12 pounds. She was thrilled. She hadn't seen the 150s in years. She decided to do the plan one more time, and found that when she recalculated her Metabolic Intervention Score, she had "graduated" to Meal Map A. After fourteen days on Meal Map A, she had lost the last 6 pounds she wanted to lose. She is now feeling awesome and looking amazing at a sleek, sexy, and strong 152 pounds. Here is what she did:

MEAL MAP B: CATHY (Recipes start on page 123.)

Week One

		A.M. WEIGHT	BREAKFAST	A.M. SNACK	LUNCH	P.M. SNACK	DINNER	OZ. OF WATER PER DAY	EXERCISE	
PART 1	MONDAY	170	CAULIFLOWER CAKES	ORANGE	*RESTAURANT: LETTUCE WRAPS WITH STEAK AND VEGETABLES* / 1 CUP STRAW-BERRIES BACK AT THE OFFICE	MANGO	CHICKEN AND BLACK BEAN TACOS	85 OUNCES	JOGGING	
	TUESDAY	168.9	QUINOA SCRAMBLE	APPLE	PINEAPPLE-GINGER CHICKEN	ASIAN PEAR	STEAK AND CABBAGE SAUTÉ WITH SWEET POTATO MASH	84 OUNCES	EPSOM SALT BATH	
	WEDNESDAY	167.7	CAULIFLOWER CAKES	ORANGE	ROAST BEEF WRAPS	MANGO	CHICKEN AND BLACK BEAN TACOS	84 OUNCES	JOGGING	
	THURSDAY	166.7	BREAKFAST SALAD	4 OUNCES NITRATE-FREE DELI TURKEY AND 8-10 OLIVES	ASPARAGUS BACON SALAD	HUMMUS AND CELERY	SAUSAGE AND ROASTED VEGGIES	83 OUNCES	REST	
	FRIDAY	166	SPINACH-MUSHROOM FRITTATA	HUMMUS AND CELERY	*RESTAURANT: 2 SUSHI ROLLS WITH TUNA AND AVOCADO, NO RICE*	4 OUNCES NITRATE-FREE JERKY AND 1/4 CUP CASHEWS	COCONUT CHICKEN	83 OUNCES	WEIGHTS	
PART 2	SATURDAY	165.1	BREAKFAST SALAD	4 OUNCES NITRATE-FREE DELI TURKEY AND 8-10 OLIVES	ASPARAGUS BACON SALAD	HUMMUS AND CELERY	SAUSAGE AND ROASTED VEGGIES	83 OUNCES	REST	
	SUNDAY	164.6	SPINACH-MUSHROOM FRITTATA	HUMMUS AND CELERY	MEXICAN CHICKEN SALAD	4 OUNCES NITRATE-FREE JERKY AND 1/4 CUP CASHEWS	COCONUT CHICKEN	82 OUNCES	EPSOM SALT BATH	

Week Two

		A.M. WEIGHT	BREAKFAST	A.M. SNACK	LUNCH	P.M. SNACK	DINNER	OZ. OF WATER PER DAY	EXERCISE	
PART 1	MONDAY	164	QUINOA SCRAMBLE	APPLE	TURKEY WRAPS	ASIAN PEAR	STEAK AND CABBAGE SAUTÉ WITH SWEET POTATO MASH	82 OUNCES	JOGGING	
	TUESDAY	162.8	CAULIFLOWER CAKES	ORANGE	PINEAPPLE-GINGER CHICKEN	MANGO	CHICKEN AND BLACK BEAN TACOS	81 OUNCES	REST	
	WEDNESDAY	161.5	QUINOA SCRAMBLE	APPLE	TURKEY WRAPS	ASIAN PEAR	STEAK AND CABBAGE SAUTÉ WITH SWEET POTATO MASH	81 OUNCES	JOGGING	
PART 2	THURSDAY	160.4	BEEFY BREAKFAST SKILLET	4 OUNCES NITRATE-FREE DELI TURKEY AND ¼ AVOCADO, SLICED	AVOCADO TUNA SALAD	HUMMUS AND CELERY	LEMON CHICKEN FETTUCCINE	80 OUNCES	EPSOM SALT BATH	
	FRIDAY	159.5	VEGGIE EGG WRAPS	HUMMUS AND CELERY	CHICKEN AND GREEN BEAN SALAD	4 OUNCES NITRATE-FREE JERKY AND ¼ CUP CASHEWS	ALMOND CRUSTED COD	80 OUNCES	WEIGHTS	
	SATURDAY	158.6	BEEFY BREAKFAST SKILLET	4 OUNCES NITRATE-FREE DELI ROAST BEEF AND 8–10 OLIVES	*RESTAURANT: 2 SUSHI ROLLS WITH TUNA AND AVOCADO, NO RICE*	4 OUNCES DELI TURKEY AND ¼ AVOCADO, SLICED	LEMON CHICKEN FETTUCCINE	79 OUNCES	REST	
	SUNDAY	158	VEGGIE EGG WRAPS	HUMMUS AND CELERY	CHICKEN AND GREEN BEAN SALAD	4 OUNCES NITRATE-FREE JERKY AND ¼ CUP CASHEWS	ALMOND CRUSTED COD	79 OUNCES	EPSOM SALT BATH	

A s you can see from Cathy's meal map, she only had two breakfasts for Part 1 over the course of the fourteen days. She found two breakfasts she liked, and alternated them. She has a busy morning with her kids, so she could make both recipes in large batches before she started the fourteen days and freeze them. For Part 2, breakfasts included two recipes for week 1 and two more recipes for week 2, which she also prepared ahead. This way, she could get up in the morning, eat her breakfast, then make breakfast for her family and get them off to school and work. She chose snacks and lunches that were quick to make, and even went out to lunch three times while staying on plan.

For dinner, she chose recipes she knew her whole family would like. She prepared enough to repeat one Part 1 recipe and two Part 2 recipes during each week, but never had any dinner more than twice. She made enough ahead of time for her own meals and her family's, and everybody loved her homemade dinners (especially the Coconut Chicken and the Lemon Chicken Fettuccine, both of which got rave reviews).

You can copy Cathy, or go your own way, as long as you stick to Meal Map B and the food list on page 56. Use this blank meal map to plan your week ahead or to keep track as you go, whichever best fits your schedule and inclinations. Don't forget to track your weight, exercise, and water. Keep track of everything on this blank meal map. A reminder of your exercise plan is located after your blank meal map. (If you are doing Meal Map A or C, use the form on page 77 or 100, respectively.)

Meal Map B (Metabolic Intervention Score 7 to 9)

Week One—Part 1

		A.M. WEIGHT	BREAKFAST	A.M. SNACK	LUNCH	P.M. SNACK	DINNER	OZ. OF WATER PER DAY	EXERCISE
	MONDAY		RECIPE: OR 1 P: 2 V: 1 F: 1 G OR CC:	1 F:	RECIPE: OR 1 P: 2 V: 1 F:	1 F:	RECIPE: OR 1 P: 2 V: 1 CC:		
PART 1	TUESDAY		RECIPE: OR 1 P: 2 V: 1 F: 1 G OR CC:	1 F:	RECIPE: OR 1 P: 2 V: 1 F:	1 F:	RECIPE: OR 1 P: 2 V: 1 CC:		
	WEDNESDAY		RECIPE: OR 1 P: 2 V: 1 F: 1 G OR CC:	1 F:	RECIPE: OR 1 P: 2 V: 1 F:	1 F:	RECIPE: OR 1 P: 2 V: 1 CC:		

KEY: P = Protein V = Veggie F = Fruit CC = Complex Carb G = Grain-Based Carb HF = Healthy Fat and Oils

	A.M. WEIGHT	BREAKFAST	A.M. SNACK	LUNCH	P.M. SNACK	DINNER	OZ. OF WATER PER DAY	EXERCISE
THURSDAY		RECIPE: OR 2 P: 1 V: 1 HF:	1 P: 1 HF:	RECIPE: OR 1 P: 2 V: 1 HF:	1 P: 1 HF:	RECIPE: OR 1 P: 2 V: 1 HF:		
FRIDAY		RECIPE: OR 2 P: 1 V: 1 HF:	1 P: 1 HF:	RECIPE: OR 1 P: 2 V: 1 HF:	1 P: 1 HF:	RECIPE: OR 1 P: 2 V: 1 HF:		
SATURDAY		RECIPE: OR 2 P: 1 V: 1 HF:	1 P: 1 HF:	RECIPE: OR 1 P: 2 V: 1 HF:	1 P: 1 HF:	RECIPE: OR 1 P: 2 V: 1 HF:		
SUNDAY		RECIPE: OR 2 P: 1 V: 1 HF:	1 P: 1 HF:	RECIPE: OR 1 P: 2 V: 1 HF:	1 P: 1 HF:	RECIPE: OR 1 P: 2 V: 1 HF:		

PART 2

KEY: P = Protein V = Veggie F = Fruit CC = Complex Carb G = Grain-Based Carb HF = Healthy Fat and Oils

Meal Map B (Metabolic Intervention Score 7 to 9)

Week Two—Part 1

	A.M. WEIGHT	BREAKFAST	A.M. SNACK	LUNCH	P.M. SNACK	DINNER	OZ. OF WATER PER DAY	EXERCISE
MONDAY		RECIPE: OR 1 P: 2 V: 1 F: 1 G OR CC:	1 F:	RECIPE: OR 1 P: 2 V: 1 F:	1 F:	RECIPE: OR 1 P: 2 V: 1 CC:		
PART 1 **TUESDAY**		RECIPE: OR 1 P: 2 V: 1 F: 1 G OR CC:	1 F:	RECIPE: OR 1 P: 2 V: 1 F:	1 F:	RECIPE: OR 1 P: 2 V: 1 CC:		
WEDNESDAY		RECIPE: OR 1 P: 2 V: 1 F: 1 G OR CC:	1 F:	RECIPE: OR 1 P: 2 V: 1 F:	1 F:	RECIPE: OR 1 P: 2 V: 1 CC:		

KEY: P = Protein V = Veggie F = Fruit CC = Complex Carb G = Grain-Based Carb HF = Healthy Fat and Oils

Meal Map B

Week Two—Part 2

	A.M. WEIGHT	BREAKFAST	A.M. SNACK	LUNCH	P.M. SNACK	DINNER	OZ. OF WATER PER DAY	EXERCISE
THURSDAY		RECIPE: OR 2 P: 1 V: 1 HF:	1 P: 1 HF:	RECIPE: OR 1 P: 2 V: 1 HF:	1 P: 1 HF:	RECIPE: OR 1 P: 2 V: 1 HF:		
FRIDAY		RECIPE: OR 2 P: 1 V: 1 HF:	1 P: 1 HF:	RECIPE: OR 1 P: 2 V: 1 HF:	1 P: 1 HF:	RECIPE: OR 1 P: 2 V: 1 HF:		
SATURDAY		RECIPE: OR 2 P: 1 V: 1 HF:	1 P: 1 HF:	RECIPE: OR 1 P: 2 V: 1 HF:	1 P: 1 HF:	RECIPE: OR 1 P: 2 V: 1 HF:		
SUNDAY		RECIPE: OR 2 P: 1 V: 1 HF:	1 P: 1 HF:	RECIPE: OR 1 P: 2 V: 1 HF:	1 P: 1 HF:	RECIPE: OR 1 P: 2 V: 1 HF:		

PART 2

KEY: P = Protein V = Veggie F = Fruit CC = Complex Carb G = Grain-Based Carb HF = Healthy Fat and Oils

Meal Map B Recommended Exercise

(See the list of approved cardio exercises, weight-lifting guidelines, and MIE exercises on page 60.)

- *Cardio:* 2 or 3 times per week, to raise your heart rate to between 120 and 140 beats per minute for 20 to 35 minutes for each session.
- *Weights:* 1 time per week, focusing on 3 major muscle groups for each session.
- *Metabolic Intervention Exercises:* Minimum of 1 time per week.

MEET JEANINE AND HER MEAL MAP C

Jeanine came to see me when she had just turned fifty and weighed 235 pounds. She told me she just didn't feel like herself anymore. Although she had always been curvy and technically overweight, hovering just at or below 200 pounds, she was tall and carried her weight well. She always felt pretty good about herself. But in the past year, she had gained 35 pounds, had no energy, and knew from her increasingly irregular cycle that menopause was imminent. Suddenly her body was changing shape practically before her eyes. She said her hourglass figure was shifting and she felt less like a bombshell and more like a balloon. She was bloated, and even suddenly developed cellulite on her upper arms and upper torso, something she had never had before. While her husband didn't seem to notice, she noticed, and felt uncomfortable most of the time. She said her stomach felt bloated, her thighs chafed, and her arms wobbled. "This is not me," she told me. "I feel like I'm hidden inside this bloated body and I just want to get out."

I explained that she was likely experiencing hormone-based weight gain, a common issue at her age, but that she was not fated to keep those extra 35 pounds for life. She just needed metabolism repair, and the Metabolism Revolution was the doorway to regaining her energy and a body she felt good about. We talked about her ideal weight, and she decided she would feel much better and be healthier if she could get back down closer to 180 pounds—but that felt like a long way to go. I told her that losing 14 pounds in fourteen days could kick-start that longer weight loss journey, and she was all in.

We calculated her Metabolic Intervention Score and saw that she would benefit most from Meal Map C. We pulled out a blank meal map and started planning. We flipped through the recipes, and she chose the ones she liked the best and that she thought her husband and daughter would also enjoy. She also told me they had an unbreakable Friday-night family restaurant night. How would she navigate that? We talked about how she could choose the restaurant, look at the menu ahead of time, and call ahead to be sure her meal would comply with her needs. "Tell them you are on a special nutrition plan and you need their help in staying compliant," I said. "Good restaurants will be happy to help you."

Next I explained how she needed to be drinking half her body weight in ounces of water. Jeanine wasn't sure she could drink 118 ounces of water every day, but I reminded her this was less than a gallon, and I told her I had clients who easily drank a gallon of water every day to help their bodies remove all those fat-soluble toxins that are released when fat burns away. She said she liked a brand of water that came in 33.8-ounce bottles. We did the math and figured out that 3½ of these bottles per day would meet her requirement, so she bought four cases of this brand of water online and kept them in her garage. Every night she pulled out three or four bottles and put them in the refrigerator for the next day.

Next we talked about exercise. Jeanine said she used to walk and hike outdoors and loved it, but as she was getting older, she was having more aches and pains and hadn't been doing much of anything. We discovered that a brisk walk got her heart rate right up into the 125- to 140-bpm range, so that was sufficient exercise for her at her current fitness level. She also had a gym membership that she was paying for but never used. She told me they not only had weight machines and a free personal trainer but also an infrared sauna and a water massage bed. She scheduled two days per week to meet with the trainer and target some major muscle groups, and then another two days when she could go just for the sauna or the water massage bed. She loved that she didn't have to pay even one dollar more than she was already paying to add in her MIEs, and she was finally making use of that gym membership she had been feeling so guilty about.

Jeanine chose to start on a Monday, after her water bottles arrived and she had bought, prepared, and frozen many of her dinners. On both Fridays, when her family eagerly awaited their restaurant night, Jeanine chose a steak house everyone liked. She called ahead and asked if she could get an 8-ounce steak prepared without any added butter or oil. She wanted to save her healthy fat serving for her salad. The restaurant was very accommodating. They prepared a steak for her the way she asked, and also a nice plate of steamed vegetables and a fresh garden salad—hold the cheese and croutons—with olive oil and balsamic vinegar. Jeanine felt satisfied and full, and her daughter said she couldn't even tell she was on a "diet."

After fourteen days, Jeanine was amazed to find that she had lost not 14 but *15 pounds*. This can sometimes happen with people who have a lot of weight to lose. Best of all, she felt great. The lower her weight went, the less she felt aches, pains, and menopausal symptoms. She had energy, she was loving getting back to the gym and taking walks outdoors with her dog, and she was even feeling sexy again. "My waist is emerging," she said. She decided to do the plan two more times, for a total of three rounds, and then go on the Fast Metabolism Diet until she got to her goal weight. "This is my new life," she said. And she looks reborn. Here's what she did:

Meal Map C: JEANINE (Recipes start on page 123.)
Week One

		A.M. WEIGHT	BREAKFAST	A.M. SNACK	LUNCH	P.M. SNACK	DINNER	OZ. OF WATER PER DAY	EXERCISE
PART 1	MONDAY	235	TROPICAL BREAKFAST BOWL	1 CUP KIWI	AHI TUNA WITH MANGO SALAD	2 CUPS CHERRIES	MEXICAN ZUCCHINI BOWL	118 OUNCES	WALKING
	TUESDAY	233.5	VERY VEGGIE HASH AND APPLE SLICES	1 CUP ASIAN PEAR	VERY BERRY CHICKEN SALAD	2 CUPS ORANGES	SHRIMP SKILLET	117 OUNCES	WEIGHTS AT GYM
	WEDNESDAY	232.3	TROPICAL BREAKFAST BOWL	1 CUP KIWI	STUFFED ACORN SQUASH	1 CUP ASIAN PEAR	LEMON SALMON WITH WILD RICE	116 OUNCES	INFARED SAUNA
PART 2	THURSDAY	230.9	BREAKFAST COLLARD WRAP	1/2 CUP HUMMUS AND CELERY	FAJITA-STUFFED CHICKEN	4 OUNCES NITRATE-FREE DELI TURKEY WITH 1/4 AVOCADO, SLICED	NUT-CRUSTED CHICKEN	115 OUNCES	WALKING
	FRIDAY	229.6	PORTOBELLO MUSHROOM BAKE	4 OUNCES JERKY AND 1/4 CUP CASHEWS	KALE SKILLET	1/2 CUP HUMMUS AND CELERY	RESTAURANT MEAL: STEAK, STEAMED VEGETABLES, SALAD WITH OLIVE OIL AND BALSAMIC VINEGAR	115 OUNCES	WEIGHTS AT GYM
	SATURDAY	228.7	PORTOBELLO MUSHROOM BAKE	4 OUNCES NITRATE-FREE DELI TURKEY WITH 8-10 OLIVES	FAJITA-STUFFED CHICKEN	4 OUNCES BEEF JERKY AND 8-10 OLIVES	SPAGHETTI SQUASH FRITTATA	114 OUNCES	WALKING
	SUNDAY	228	BREAKFAST COLLARD WRAP	4 OUNCES TURKEY JERKY AND 1/4 CUP CASHEWS	SPICY TIPS	4 OUNCES BACON CHIPS AND 1/4 CUP GUACAMOLE	GINGER-LIME SALMON	114 OUNCES	WATER MASSAGE BED

Meal Map of JEANINE

Week Two

		A.M. WEIGHT	BREAKFAST	A.M. SNACK	LUNCH	P.M. SNACK	DINNER	OZ. OF WATER PER DAY	EXERCISE
PART 1	MONDAY	226.9	APPLE SLAW BOWL	1 CUP CHERRIES	AHI WITH MANGO SALSA	2 CUPS KIWI	LEMON-TURMERIC QUINOA WITH PORK MEDALLION	113 OUNCES	WALKING
	TUESDAY	225.8	TROPICAL FRUIT BOWL	1 CUP ASIAN PEAR	VERY BERRY CHICKEN SALAD	2 CUPS STRAWBERRIES	LEMON SALMON WITH WILD RICE	113 OUNCES	WEIGHTS AT GYM
	WEDNESDAY	225	VERY VEGGIE HASH	1 CUP BLACKBERRIES	STUFFED ACORN SQUASH	2 CUPS ORANGES	MEXICAN ZUCCHINI BOWL	113 OUNCES	INFARED SAUNA
PART 2	THURSDAY	223.7	BREAKFAST BACON COLLARD WRAP	4 OUNCES NITRATE-FREE DELI ROAST BEEF AND 8-10 OLIVES	KALE SKILLET	4 OUNCES BACON CHIPS AND 1/4 CUP GUACAMOLE	NUT-CRUSTED CHICKEN	112 OUNCES	WALKING
	FRIDAY	222.5	CAULIFLOWER "RICE" BOWL	1/2 CUP HUMMUS (CONTAINS LEGUMES AND SEED BUTTER) AND CELERY (FREE FOOD)	SPICY TIPS	4 OUNCES BEEF JERKY AND 8-10 OLIVES	*RESTAURANT MEAL: STEAK, STEAMED VEGETABLES, SALAD WITH OLIVE OIL AND BALSAMIC VINEGAR*	111 OUNCES	WEIGHTS AT GYM
	SATURDAY	221.3	BREAKFAST BACON COLLARD WRAP	4 OUNCES NITRATE-FREE DELI TURKEY AND 1/4 AVOCADO, SLICED	KALE SKILLET	1/2 CUP HUMMUS AND CELERY	GINGER-LIME SALMON	111 OUNCES	WALKING
	SUNDAY	220	PORTOBELLO MUSHROOM BAKE	1/2 CUP HUMMUS AND CELERY STICKS	FAJITA-STUFFED CHICKEN	4 OUNCES BACON CHIPS AND 1/4 CUP GUACAMOLE	SPAGHETTI SQUASH STIR-FRY	110 OUNCES	WATER MASSAGE BED

A s you can see from Jeanine's Meal Map C, she really enjoyed a Tropical Breakfast Bowl for breakfast during Part 1. She had it twice during the first week and once during the second week. Lunches were the same during Part 1 for weeks 1 and 2, and the same for Part 2 but in a different order. For dinner, she made a total of four dinners for Part 1 and four dinners for Part 2. She also successfully navigated her Friday-night family restaurant night during both weeks while staying completely on plan.

You can eat just like Jeanine ate, or make your own choices, as long as you stick to Meal Map C and the food list on page 56. Use this blank meal map to plan your week ahead or to keep track as you go, whichever best fits your schedule and inclinations. Don't forget to track your weight, exercise, and water. Your blank meal map is your central organizer, and a reminder of your exercise plan is located after your blank meal map. (If you are doing Meal Map A or B, use the form on page 77 or 88, respectively.)

Meal Map C (Metabolic Intervention Score 6 or less)

Week One—Part 1

	A.M. WEIGHT	BREAKFAST	A.M. SNACK	LUNCH	P.M. SNACK	DINNER	OZ. OF WATER PER DAY	EXERCISE
MONDAY		RECIPE: OR 2 P: 2 V: 1 F: 1 G OR CC:	1 F:	RECIPE: OR 1 P: 2 V: 2 F:	2 F:	RECIPE: OR 2 P: 2 V: 1 CC:		
TUESDAY		RECIPE: OR 2 P: 2 V: 1 F: 1 G OR CC:	1 F:	RECIPE: OR 1 P: 2 V: 2 F:	2 F:	RECIPE: OR 2 P: 2 V: 1 CC:		
WEDNESDAY		RECIPE: OR 2 P: 2 V: 1 F: 1 G OR CC:	1 F:	RECIPE: OR 1 P: 2 V: 2 F:	2 F:	RECIPE: OR 2 P: 2 V: 1 CC:		

PART 1

KEY: P = Protein V = Veggie F = Fruit CC = Complex Carb G = Grain-Based Carb HF = Healthy Fat and Oils

Week One—Part 2

	A.M. WEIGHT	BREAKFAST	A.M. SNACK	LUNCH	P.M. SNACK	DINNER	OZ. OF WATER PER DAY	EXERCISE
THURSDAY		RECIPE: OR 2 P: 2 V: 1 HF:	1 P: 1 HF:	RECIPE: OR 2 P: 2 V: 1 HF:	1 P: 1 HF:	RECIPE: OR 2 P: 2 V: 1 HF:		
FRIDAY		RECIPE: OR 2 P: 2 V: 1 HF:	1 P: 1 HF:	RECIPE: OR 2 P: 2 V: 1 HF:	1 P: 1 HF:	RECIPE: OR 2 P: 2 V: 1 HF:		
PART 2 **SATURDAY**		RECIPE: OR 2 P: 2 V: 1 HF:	1 P: 1 HF:	RECIPE: OR 2 P: 2 V: 1 HF:	1 P: 1 HF:	RECIPE: OR 2 P: 2 V: 1 HF:		
SUNDAY		RECIPE: OR 2 P: 2 V: 1 HF:	1 P: 1 HF:	RECIPE: OR 2 P: 2 V: 1 HF:	1 P: 1 HF:	RECIPE: OR 2 P: 2 V: 1 HF:		

KEY: P = Protein V = Veggie F = Fruit CC = Complex Carb G = Grain-Based Carb HF = Healthy Fat and Oils

Meal Map C (Metabolic Intervention Score 6 or less)

Week Two—Part 1

	A.M. WEIGHT	BREAKFAST	A.M. SNACK	LUNCH	P.M. SNACK	DINNER	OZ. OF WATER PER DAY	EXERCISE
MONDAY		RECIPE: OR 2 P: 2 V: 1 F: 1 G OR CC:	1 F:	RECIPE: OR 1 P: 2 V: 2 F:	2 F:	RECIPE: OR 2 P: 2 V: 1 CC:		
PART 1 TUESDAY		RECIPE: OR 2 P: 2 V: 1 F: 1 G OR CC:	1 F:	RECIPE: OR 1 P: 2 V: 2 F:	2 F:	RECIPE: OR 2 P: 2 V: 1 CC:		
WEDNESDAY		RECIPE: OR 2 P: 2 V: 1 F: 1 G OR CC:	1 F:	RECIPE: OR 1 P: 2 V: 2 F:	2 F:	RECIPE: OR 2 P: 2 V: 1 CC:		

KEY: P = Protein V = Veggie F = Fruit CC = Complex Carb G = Grain-Based Carb HF = Healthy Fat and Oils

Week Two—Part 2

	A.M. WEIGHT	BREAKFAST	A.M. SNACK	LUNCH	P.M. SNACK	DINNER	OZ. OF WATER PER DAY	EXERCISE
THURSDAY		RECIPE: OR 2 P: 2 V: 1 HF:	1 P: 1 HF:	RECIPE: OR 2 P: 2 V: 1 HF:	1 P: 1 HF:	RECIPE: OR 2 P: 2 V: 1 HF:		
FRIDAY		RECIPE: OR 2 P: 2 V: 1 HF:	1 P: 1 HF:	RECIPE: OR 2 P: 2 V: 1 HF:	1 P: 1 HF:	RECIPE: OR 2 P: 2 V: 1 HF:		
PART 2 **SATURDAY**		RECIPE: OR 2 P: 2 V: 1 HF:	1 P: 1 HF:	RECIPE: OR 2 P: 2 V: 1 HF:	1 P: 1 HF:	RECIPE: OR 2 P: 2 V: 1 HF:		
SUNDAY		RECIPE: OR 2 P: 2 V: 1 HF:	1 P: 1 HF:	RECIPE: OR 2 P: 2 V: 1 HF:	1 P: 1 HF:	RECIPE: OR 2 P: 2 V: 1 HF:		

KEY: P = Protein V = Veggie F = Fruit CC = Complex Carb G = Grain-Based Carb HF = Healthy Fat and Oils

Meal Map C Recommended Exercise

(See the list of approved cardio exercises, weight-lifting guidelines, and MIE exercises on page 60.)

- *Cardio:* 2 or 3 times per week, to raise your heart rate to between 120 and 140 beats per minute for 20 to 35 minutes for each session.
- *Weights:* 2 times per week, focusing on 3 major muscle groups for each session.
- *Metabolic Intervention Exercises:* Minimum of 2 times per week.

5

YEAH, BUT WHAT IF . . . ?: METABOLISM REVOLUTION FAQS

One of the things I love most about the clients who come to my clinic and my member community is that they are all full of so many smart, savvy questions. I've collected these frequently asked questions from my clients who have been on the Metabolism Revolution program—maybe they're questions you have, too. I hope you will find yourself in some of these questions and that my answers will help inspire you and keep you going. If you think of something that isn't on this list, please join my robust community and become part of our active online chats. Ask me, ask my team, ask the other members. Become part of our challenges, our recipe contests, and our mutual support and inspiration. We are all there to support one another, share our experiences, and cheer one another on. My goal is that you and I will be friends for a long, long time. Now, here are my answers to those frequently asked questions.

GENERAL QUESTIONS ABOUT THE METABOLISM REVOLUTION PLAN

Q: I'm not convinced that men and women should share the same ideal weight range. Are you sure that's right?

A: I've already addressed this briefly, but the idea that men always weigh more than women, or women always less than men, is antiquated. If you knew how much some of my clients *actually weighed*, you would feel a lot better about yourself. If I have a male client and a female client who are both 5 feet 5 inches tall, it's a crapshoot who will weigh more—the man with his muscles or the woman with her hips and boobs. Some men don't have all that much muscle. Some women are well-endowed. You can't stereotype bodies or health. The weight ranges I provide in this program, when you are calculating your ideal weight on page 28, are *ranges* because they make allowances for these kinds of individual differences. So yes—they share an ideal weight range. But they may not share the same ideal weight goal. That's personal.

Q: I've been on the Fast Metabolism Diet and lost a lot of weight rapidly, and you have said that FMD is a rapid weight loss diet. If I already have your twenty-eight-day rapid weight loss diet, why would I do this fourteen-day rapid weight loss diet?

A: That is an excellent question, and I'm sure many long-time FMD-ers are wondering the same thing. FMD *is* a rapid weight loss diet, but Metabolism Revolution is a shorter, faster-acting rapid weight loss diet. On FMD, you can lose up to 20 pounds in twenty-eight days, but over a shorter period of time, you can actually sustain up to a 1-pound-per-day weight loss, which is even more rapid.

However, both FMD and Metabolism Revolution are based on a unifying concept of "confuse it to lose it," a process of changing the macronutrient ratios throughout the week. For some people, fourteen days and 14 pounds is all they will ever need, but for others with bigger weight loss goals, Metabolism Revolution is a great way to begin, and FMD could be a tool to use later, as weight loss progresses. You can do the Metabolism Revolution plan up to three times in succession to lose more than 14 pounds, but after that, if my clients are still working on weight loss, I like them to switch it up and try something else. Some people have 75 to 100 pounds or more to lose, so it's great to have options. Changing it up can shake you out of plateaus over the longer term, and this is a bigger-picture version of "confuse it to lose it."

> **Q:** I work out a lot/teach fitness classes/am training for a marathon, and I can't/don't want to change my training schedule. Do I need to adjust this diet in any way?

A: Yes, but the adjustment is easy and pleasant. If you are doing an exercise that makes your heart rate go over 120 beats per minute (bpm) for longer than 10 minutes, then you should add a fruit before your exercise session, no matter what part of the week you are on. Also, if you are exercising more than four days per week with a sustained heart rate over 120 bpm for longer than 10 minutes, you need to add an additional serving of protein on every day that you do this over four days. This protein serving should be with either breakfast or lunch.

Note that this system accounts for variations in fitness. If you are very fit, it will take a lot more exercise to get you up to 120 bpm and keep you there for over 10 minutes, so be sure to measure your heart rate to confirm that you need that extra fruit or protein serving. If you are less fit but exercising vigorously, you are more likely to need this extra nutritional boost until your fitness increases.

Q: I'm pregnant/a nursing mother. Can I do this plan?

A: I don't suggest weight loss during pregnancy, so this is not a plan for pregnant women. Remember that weight loss promotes detoxification, and pregnancy is not the time to help your body release fat-soluble toxins at an aggressive rate. However, this is an excellent diet for those who are planning to become pregnant soon. You can get extra weight off and clear toxins from your system, which will create a more beneficial internal environment for pregnancy.

If you are nursing, you are probably already losing weight quickly, but if you aren't, your primary goal should not be weight loss. Hydration and rest are king (or queen). Drink all your water, sleep enough at night, and don't feel bad about napping. Nutritionally, the goal is to keep milk quantity and quality high. That being said, you can do this program while you are nursing, *if* you:

1. Add two servings of healthy fats per day into the first part of your week, at any meal or snack, and
2. Add two servings of fruit per day into the second half of the week, at any meal or snack.

Remember, this is *only if you are nursing.* Once your baby is weaned, go back to the plan as it is written.

Q: I have a really active job (like construction) and I burn a lot of calories. Do I need to eat more?

A: Not necessarily. As long as this is not a new job and your body is already conditioned for the position, this plan provides tons of nutrients to support your high level of physicality. Your body has already regulated its metabolic dysfunction to your current level of physical stress, so to effect rapid weight loss, you need to do something different. However, I don't want you losing more than 1 pound per day when you are being this physical, so if you find that you are losing more than that on this diet, then you can make one of these two changes: *either* double your snack portions *or* add a third snack, either before breakfast or at the end of the day.

Q: I'm in sales and constantly have to entertain clients at restaurants and bars. Can I make this plan work for me?

A: Absolutely. Many of my clients are working professionals who travel a lot, are on tour or on the road, or have busy active lives that take them out of their home kitchens frequently. My best advice is to plan ahead, plan ahead, plan ahead. Don't get caught up in an unexpected food situation—expect anything. Let's make a date—me, you, your calendar, and a cup of hot herbal tea. We're going to plan this out so you know exactly what's happening on any given night and what you will do in any situation. Specifically, here are my best tips for you:

1. Try to be proactive in selecting the restaurants.
2. Get the menu ahead of time. Most restaurants have their menus online.

3. Call ahead to tell the restaurant you are on a special nutrition plan and ask them about replacement foods or preparations. Some restaurants charge for substitutions if you ask them on the spot, but I have never seen a restaurant charge one of my clients when they called ahead to arrange their meals.

4. Bring food on the road so you aren't relying only on restaurants for your nutrition when you travel. Make tons of the jerky recipe and vacuum seal it for travel, along with raw nuts and seeds.

5. When the drinks are free-flowing, remember this plan only lasts for fourteen days, and for now, you are on the wagon—a club soda with lime is all the cocktail you need. The best response I've heard to belly-to-the-bar peer pressure is to tell your colleagues you are on "an intense nutrient-infusion plan," so you can't indulge tonight. They will know you are a badass, and they may even follow your lead.

Q: Can kids do this diet or safely eat the food I am making for myself?

A: Every recipe on this plan is perfectly healthy for children, and may contain more nutrient-dense foods than they were eating before. This is not "diet food." It is good, whole, real food. Your kids will probably really love some of these recipes, which may become new family favorites. That being said, they can eat larger portions if they are active, and they can add other healthy foods to this diet.

If you are hoping to use this diet to help your kids lose weight, I will tell you that I never use the term *weight loss* with kids. When children are still growing, the most important thing for them is to establish healthy and active metabolic pathways that will serve them well for the rest of their lives. Kids go through phases of growth and rest, and in the presence of a nutrient-infused diet, weight issues tend to work themselves out. Because we are focusing on establishing those metabolic pathways, children who are still growing need more fruit than this plan provides. For young people eating this plan, add more fruit, specifically in Part 2, when you would not be having fruit as an adult seeking rapid weight loss. Kids should be having five servings of fruit *per day, every day,* which means fruit with every meal and snack, whether or not you are having it, too. This also applies to teenagers (see the next question).

> **Q:** I'm a teenager with 50 pounds to lose. Do I need to alter this diet in any way?

A: The teenage years are an incredible time to work on enhancing and maximizing your metabolism. Your hormones are starting to navigate their very own pathways, and whole fruits are critical during this time of your life. I don't like to emphasize weight loss for kids, but for older teenagers who want to get to a healthy weight before adulthood, the Metabolism Revolution is a good place to start. However, when you apply the program, I want you to make this one very important change: Make sure you get five full servings of fruits every day, whether it is called for in the basic program or not.

Whole fruits are *critical* during this time in your life. Let's say you are doing Meal Map B. In Part 1, your day includes four fruit servings. I want you to add another one, with dinner, or by doubling one of your other fruit servings. In Part 2, when the diet doesn't include any fruit servings, I want you to add one serving with every meal and snack. This *will not compromise your weight loss goals.* Because you are a teenager, your metabolism is not yet set the way an adult's would be, and this fruit is crucial for making sure that when your metabolism does get more permanently established, it does so in a way that benefits your health and weight. Even when you are not on this diet, I strongly recommend eating five servings of fruit every day.

I also want to give you a special caution when you are calculating your ideal body weight. Once you have calculated your ideal minimum and maximum, I want you to select your ideal goal weight from somewhere in the middle of that range. I don't want you to obsess about hitting the very lowest number. This is not a time of life to "diet" in a traditional manner. If you do that now, listen to me when I tell you that *you will be doing it for the rest of your life.* This is a fun time to reset your metabolism so you can have a fast one in your thirties, forties, fifties, and beyond. I know you're probably not thinking about retirement right now, or your waistline during menopause, but trust me—many of my clients would kill to go back in time and create healthy hormone pathways in their teens. They look back on that time and regret that they didn't know. You have a huge advantage here, so follow this program with the added five servings of whole fruits every day, and you will be doing yourself a favor for the rest of your life.

Q: How do I feed my family on this diet? Should they eat what I'm eating if they don't want to lose weight?

A: Your family can certainly eat the same meals you are eating on this diet. In fact, my clients find that when they feed these meals to their families, the whole family's health improves because the meals are more nutrient-dense than what they were all eating before. For those who aren't trying to lose weight or repair their metabolisms, portion sizes aren't as crucial. Let them go back for seconds—a lot of these recipes become family favorites, and people are always going back for more. Also, they can also make additions to the meals, such as adding more protein, vegetables, or complex carbohydrates, or sprinkling their meals with cheese or pickle slices or whatever they like. Just make these options available at the table rather than at the stove. That way, you are all sharing a meal, but at the same time, you can easily structure your meal the way you need it, while still giving other family members the freedom to adapt their meals to their preferences.

When kids make these meals their own, they expand their palates and their micronutrient consumption without even noticing they are eating "healthy foods," and everyone starts feeling better. And don't worry about other family members not getting enough calories. These meals are strategically designed to unlock stored fat, but in people who don't have excess stored fat or metabolic dysfunction, the meals won't have that effect. They will simply deliver amazing nutrients to build muscle, bone, skin, hair, and nails. It's real food, designed to nourish any and every body.

Q: I have limited or no mobility, and I can't do the exercise plan. Can I just skip it? Does that mean I have to change the food plan in any way?

A: No, don't skip exercise. But "exercise" doesn't mean you have to run a marathon or take up kickboxing. If you have mobility issues, please select MIEs—passive or supported exercise options—in place of cardio and weight lifting, to the extent necessary for your needs. These count as exercise, too. You'll notice that in the exercise plan, I have included such activities as infrared sauna, massage, dry skin brushing, physical therapy, hot baths, Epsom salt baths, and acupuncture. As long as you are doing something that stimulates your circulation and blood flow at least three times per week, you are exercising.

I provide lots of options, so your choices don't have to be expensive. Sometimes you can find coupons for free introductory massages or infrared sauna sessions or acupuncture visits. Look for opportunities, specials, coupons, and promotions during the fourteen days, especially for things you've never tried before. You may find a favorite new therapy. Other things like baths are cheap, and you can often find Epsom salts and dry brushes at the dollar store.

A word about physical therapy: I think physical therapy is one of the most underutilized forms of exercise available. If you can get a prescription for physical therapy from your doctor, please do so. If you only get so many visits per year, this is the time to use them.

> **Q:** I missed/had to skip my cardio/weight-lifting session for the week. Can I make up for it?

A: Absolutely. While exercise does many important metabolism-enhancing things for you, I know that sometimes life happens and you end up missing a session (or three). In those instances, you can always replace a cardio or weight-lifting workout with an MIE. This will give you many of the benefits of exercise, including stress relief and increased circulation. Find a list of MIEs on page 63.

> **Q:** I've had gastric bypass surgery. Do I need to modify this plan?

A: Yes, typically those who have had gastric bypass surgery can't consume the large portions of protein, vegetables, and fruit called for in this plan. But you *can* still do the plan. When I have clients who have gone through this, we typically divide the meals into eight to ten smaller meals, so you will be eating more frequently but in smaller amounts, which gives your body the chance to properly digest the food each time. There are also other ways to make nutrient-dense food less bulky and easier to digest and absorb. You can cook and puree vegetables and fruits, and even meats. Sometimes, I do find that the size of meat protein portions is too much for those with gastric bypass. I can usually get 20 to 26 grams of protein into you with my shakes, which you can certainly try, but it's harder to get the protein this high with meat. Listen to your body, and if it's really too much, you can reduce the portions to an amount that is comfortable for you.

QUESTIONS ABOUT THE FOOD LIST AND PORTION SIZES

Q: Does iceberg lettuce count as an approved lettuce on the vegetable list?

A: Iceberg lettuce has the lowest number of micronutrients per cup of all lettuces. It is also typically an agricultural crop that has a significant amount of herbicide and pesticide applied to it. For both of these reasons, it is my least recommended lettuce. Dark green, soft lettuces typically have a better impact on overall metabolism and are more likely to stimulate weight loss.

Q: On some of your other plans, cucumbers are a free food. Why aren't they a free food on this plan?

A: Based on my personal experiences with clients, I have not selected cucumbers as a free food for the Metabolism Revolution. I have observed that when cucumbers are "free," many of my clients really go to town on them. They eat them every day, multiple times per day, to the exclusion of all the other delicious vegetables available for snacks and meals. When cucumbers are eaten chronically in this way, they lose their strategic impact, so I am doling them out purposefully to you during this program. I want you to get all their wonderful benefits without going overboard into cucumber land. But cucumbers are an excellent vegetable choice, with an incredible amount of fiber and potassium, so when I do suggest them, I hope you will enjoy them fully. (In the approved portion sizes, of course.)

Q: In the food list, you use the term *pure* to describe mustards and vinegars. What do you mean by that?

A: These condiments have a history of being loaded with sugars, honey, dextrose, and other ingredients that slow down the metabolism. If you're going to use these, you have to be a label reader and make sure that nothing fishy is in there. The nutrition label for most mustards should only list mustard seeds, vinegar, and spices as ingredients, and vinegar labels shouldn't list much more than the main ingredient for which the vinegar is named (for example, apple cider for apple cider vinegar, red wine for red wine vinegar, etc.; balsamic vinegar should list "grape must" as the first or second ingredient).

Q: Do nuts count as a protein and a fat for a snack, or do I also need to add a protein?

A: For the Metabolism Revolution, raw nuts and seeds fall into the healthy fat category. Even though they do contain protein, they do not go into the protein count for that meal or snack. This is an important distinction for my purposes for this diet. This means you will need to select a food item from the protein category to round out that requirement.

Q: For dinner with a complex carb and a protein, can I just have two servings of legumes?

A: Yes, if you do it correctly. The servings for legumes, when counted as a complex carb, are one portion, and the servings of a legume when counted as a protein are another portion. For example, for a Meal Map B Part 1 dinner, you could have ½ cup black beans for your protein and another ½ cup for your complex carbohydrate. As long as you use the appropriate portion for your meal map, you will be spot on.

Q: Why are wild rice and quinoa on the non-grain carb list? Aren't those grains?

A: Actually, they are seeds, not grains, and have a much lower starch content. You may be confused if you have read some of my other books, because in the past, I have listed these in the grain category. That was purposeful for that particular diet. For this diet, however, and for our purposes now, wild rice and quinoa should be counted as a non-grain carb, so you can have them with dinner in Part 1.

Q: Do I have to eat the grains whole, or can I have them in some easier-to-eat, quick form like spelt pretzels, sprouted-grain bread (using a compliant grain), crackers, or tortillas?

A: If you find a pure and compliant product with no additives—like pure brown rice tortillas, sprouted buckwheat bread, or those beloved spelt pretzels—then knock yourself out, as long as the product isn't adulterated with other ingredients. Again, you have to be an avid label reader.

Q: I use Meal Map C, but two servings of protein seems like a lot, especially for breakfast. How am I supposed to eat a four-egg omelet or 8 ounces of turkey sausage?

A: I selected each of the food categories based on the degree of metabolic intervention your body needs. Protein is a key player in healing the metabolism, especially for people using Meal Map C. However, you don't have to select all four servings of the same food. Mix it up. You could have two eggs and 4 ounces of nitrate-free chicken sausage or turkey bacon, for example. That being said, always listen to your body. If you really can't eat your whole meal, don't force yourself. But don't hold back because you think it will help you lose weight faster, either. With my clients, I find that big goals require big intervention.

Q: Seriously, how am I supposed to eat 4 cups of vegetables for breakfast?

A: The best way to do this is to chew, chew, chew. Oh, wait, you said "seriously." Okay then. Remember, we are activating digestive enzymes, releasing micronutrients, rebalancing hormone distribution, and stimulating release of stubborn fat, and vegetables are the key to all these very important jobs. You might not be *used to* eating vegetables for breakfast, but they are taking care of major work for you right now. They are like kindling for the fire. Still, that doesn't mean you have to choke down 4 cups of sliced cucumbers at six A.M. There are easier ways. Some people like to puree their veggies and add them to a smoothie, or even make them into a soup (soup for breakfast is common in some cultures). Or cook them up with eggs—use onions, peppers, chopped spinach, or whatever you like. When cooked, that 4 cups really shrinks down to a manageable size.

Q: I find it really hard to drink all that water. Any tips?

A: My community is always offering ideas about how to get in all that water (which is so worthwhile). Some say they put all the ounces they need today into a pitcher first thing in the morning or the night before. Then they don't have to keep track—they just keep pouring glasses from the pitcher until it's empty. You can keep this in the refrigerator or not, depending on whether you like your water cold or at room temperature. Others know exactly how many water bottles they will need, and bring them to the office. One community member keeps four tokens and a small dish by the sink. Every time she fills her 24-ounce bottle from her reverse-osmosis tap, she puts one token in the dish. When they are all in the dish, she's done. Another uses quarters and pays herself for every bottle, and another puts six bangle bracelets on her right wrist and moves one to her left wrist every time she refills her water bottle. I have such ingenious community members.

Q: Does zucchini count as a squash?

A: Yes, zucchini is a summer squash.

Q: Can I have jicama?

A: I have purposefully not added jicama to the Metabolism Revolution. However, you will notice that it is on the Fast Metabolism 4 Life food list, so you can look forward to eating jicama when you are on the maintenance plan.

Q: All that fruit is upsetting my stomach. Should I really be eating six servings a day? That seems like a lot.

A: Again, above all, listen to your body, but also consider that the amount of fruit isn't the problem. It might be the *type* of fruit. Try selecting different fruits. Another way to make fruit even more digestible is to cook it gently on the stove with a little water. Also, make sure that when you eat, you try to create a relaxed environment and chew each bite fully to stimulate the release of digestive enzymes. Nothing causes stomach upset like stressing out while you eat.

Q: Why can't I have tomatoes? I can't imagine my life without salsa and your famous chili.

A: In many of my plans, you will find tomatoes in a variety of decadent and delicious recipes. But nothing says you have to eat them every day of your life, and for the Metabolism Revolution, I have strategically pulled this fruit/vegetable to allow other foods to shine. Never fear—we are going to be cooking together for a long, long time, and when you are on the 4 Life plan to maintain your weight loss (or if you are trying some of my other plans, like the Fast Metabolism Diet), tomatoes are A-OK.

Q: I love coconut milk in my herbal tea/on my oatmeal. Can this count as a healthy fat?

A: I've purposely left nut milks, including coconut milk, out of this plan. For now, use the whole coconut, raw, or coconut oil in your oatmeal. Or try other raw nuts or seeds instead. Your body can extract sugar more quickly and easily from nut milks like coconut milk than it can from the actual coconut (or nut) itself. If you are looking for a way to make your oatmeal less thick, just prepare it with additional water. The only exception I allow is if you puree your own fresh coconut meat, in the appropriate portion for the appropriate serving, with as much water as you want. This homemade "coconut milk" will be free of additives and less willing to release its sugars because it contains all the natural fiber of the coconut meat, which store-bought coconut milk does not. I have one client who loves cream in her coffee, and she prepare batches of her own homemade coconut milk, pours it into ice cube trays, and freezes it. Every morning, she pops one into her herbal tea. Genius.

> **Q:** I want to do the food plan rather than the supported plan, but are there ways to occasionally substitute one of your shakes for any of the meals or snacks? Sometimes this would be really convenient.

A: You can absolutely do this. You can use my Metabolism Meal Replacement shakes once a week on that one really busy day you always have, or up to twice a day every day as a replacement for any breakfast or lunch. They are food-based and micronutrient-focused products meant to support you in times of need. Some of my clients run out the door with a shake every morning, and others use them when they travel. I tend to do a little bit of both of those, and most of my clients fall somewhere in the middle, too. So, while there is a Super-Simple Supported Plan that uses the shakes twice a day for the truly time-crunched or cooking-averse, you can always choose to cook when you want and substitute a shake for any breakfast or lunch during a day when you run out of time, energy, or clean foods to eat.

Q: I know coffee isn't on the list, but are there any healthy substitutes I could have during the fourteen days, like caffeine-free herbal tea or a grain-based coffee substitute like Pero or Dandy Blend?

A: I do discourage coffee. In fact, I'm downright against it, for many reasons (in particular, see "The Elephant in the Room" on page 58). But that doesn't mean you can't enjoy a warm cuppa. Herbs and spices are on your free food list, which means a cup of herbal tea made with dry or fresh herbs is just fine. Don't have real tea (black, green, or white, even decaffeinated), but there are many excellent and even therapeutic teas to try, like peppermint, ginger, chamomile, lemon, or dandelion tea, which has a roasty, coffeelike flavor and is also an excellent tonic for your liver.

If tea isn't quite right for you and you want something even more coffeelike, you could try Pero, a coffee substitute made from roasted grains. I don't encourage doing this every day, but it might help you get off coffee. Some of my community even take a week to break their coffee habit *before* starting the fourteen-day plan (or the twenty-eight-day Fast Metabolism Diet plan, or any of my other plans), because for many, that is the hardest part. Just remember that Pero and similar grain-based coffee substitutes are *not* gluten-free, so if you have celiac disease or non-celiac gluten sensitivity, you should not use these products. Also, even if you are not specifically gluten-sensitive but have other types of allergies such as inhalant or skin allergies, be aware that gluten can be a catalyst nutrient for histamine, and that could worsen your allergy symptoms. For this reason, I don't recommend grain-based coffee substitutes (or any other gluten-containing food) for anyone with any kind of allergies, whether inhalant, skin, or food.

6

METABOLISM REVOLUTION RECIPES

These Metabolism Revolution recipes are super-simple to make, so no worries about lots of prep time or cooking. All the recipes mentioned in the client meal maps from the last chapter are included here, and every recipe is adaptable to Meal Maps A, B, and C. The chapter is also divided by recipes appropriate for Parts 1 and 2. At the end of this chapter, you can find a few of my favorite "free" recipes, which you can eat on any day, at any time, and in any amount. These are perfect little treats that are fun to eat and can help keep you even more satisfied without any negative impact on your weight loss.

When preparing these recipes, find the column for your individual meal map, A, B, or C. Use the measurement under your meal map column for preparation. If the recipe serves more than one, divide your completed prepared food by the number of servings that the recipe designates. Use any additional servings to feed others, or keep in the freezer for future meals. You can also double, triple, or quadruple any recipe in this book if it serves one. This will allow you to serve others or save additional servings for later.

BREAKFASTS, PART 1

Savory Oats

SERVES 1

INGREDIENTS	MEAL MAP A	MEAL MAP B	MEAL MAP C
OLD-FASHIONED OATS*	½ CUP	½ CUP	½ CUP
FRESH THYME SPRIG	1	1	1
SEA SALT	PINCH	PINCH	PINCH
EGGS**	2	2	2
MUSHROOMS	1 CUP SLICED	2 CUPS SLICED	2 CUPS SLICED
BABY SPINACH	1 CUP	2 CUPS	2 CUPS
RED PEPPER FLAKES	PINCH	PINCH	PINCH
APPLE, CORED AND SLICED	1	1	1
TURKEY BACON,** NITRATE-FREE, COOKED	NONE	NONE	4 SLICES

1. Cook the oats according to the package instructions. Reduce the heat to low to keep the oats at a bare simmer. Add the thyme sprig and salt, stir, and cover. Leave undisturbed for at least 5 minutes, or until cooked to your desired consistency.

2. While the oatmeal is cooking, poach or fry the eggs in a nonstick pan (don't use oil), and sauté the mushrooms and spinach.

3. Remove the oatmeal from the heat, remove the thyme sprig, and spoon the oats into a bowl.

4. Top the oats with the eggs, mushrooms, and spinach. Garnish with the red pepper flakes and serve with the apple slices and, for Meal Map C only, turkey bacon.

*If you don't eat any grain, you may substitute any non-grain complex carb from the Metabolism Revolution Food List on page 56.

**If you don't eat any animal products, you may substitute any vegetarian protein from the Metabolism Revolution Food List on page 56.

Breakfast Hash

SERVES 1

INGREDIENTS	MEAL MAP A	MEAL MAP B	MEAL MAP C
TURKEY BACON,* NITRATE-FREE, CHOPPED	2 SLICES	2 SLICES	4 SLICES
SWEET POTATO	½ CUP DICED	½ CUP DICED	½ CUP DICED
APPLE	1 CUP DICED	1 CUP DICED	1 CUP DICED
ONION	½ CUP DICED	1 CUP DICED	1 CUP DICED
SEA SALT	¼ TEASPOON	¼ TEASPOON	½ TEASPOON
GROUND CINNAMON	¼ TEASPOON	¼ TEASPOON	¼ TEASPOON
BABY SPINACH	1 ½ CUPS	3 CUPS	3 CUPS
EGG(S)*	1	1	2

1. In a heavy medium skillet, cook the bacon over medium-high heat. When the bacon begins to brown and is halfway done, add the sweet potato. Cook, stirring, and add a little water if needed to help cook the sweet potato.

2. Once the sweet potato is getting brown and soft, add the apple and onion to the pan and stir. Reduce the heat to medium or medium-low and cover the pan. Cook for about 45 seconds to 1 minute, uncover, and stir. Add the salt and cinnamon and cook, stirring, until the mixture is nicely browned and the apple and onion have softened and lightly browned. Add the spinach and cook until wilted.

3. Remove from the pan and transfer the hash to a plate. In a nonstick skillet, fry the egg without oil (or poach it) and place it on top of the apple–sweet potato hash. Serve.

*If you don't eat any animal products, you may substitute any vegetarian protein from the Metabolism Revolution Food List on page 56.

Black Bean Scramble

SERVES 1

INGREDIENTS	MEAL MAP A	MEAL MAP B	MEAL MAP C
EGGS*	2	2	2
CANNED BLACK BEANS, DRAINED AND RINSED	1/2 CUP	1/2 CUP	1/2 CUP
GREEN BELL PEPPER	1/3 CUP CHOPPED	2/3 CUP CHOPPED	2/3 CUP CHOPPED
ONION	1/4 CUP MINCED	1/2 CUP MINCED	1/2 CUP MINCED
BABY SPINACH	1 3/4 CUPS	3 1/2 CUPS	3 1/2 CUPS
CHILI POWDER	1/4 TEASPOON	1/4 TEASPOON	1/4 TEASPOON
CAYENNE PEPPER OR RED PEPPER FLAKES	DASH	DASH	DASH
SEA SALT AND GROUND PEPPER	AS NEEDED	AS NEEDED	AS NEEDED
CANTALOUPE	1 CUP CUBED	1 CUP CUBED	1 CUP CUBED
TURKEY BACON,* NITRATE-FREE, COOKED	NONE	NONE	4 SLICES

1. In a medium nonstick skillet, combine the eggs, black beans, bell pepper, onion, spinach, chili powder, cayenne, and salt and black pepper to taste.

2. Cook over medium heat until the eggs are cooked through.

3. Serve with the cantaloupe and, for Meal Map C only, turkey bacon on the side.

*If you don't eat any animal products, you may substitute any vegetarian protein from the Metabolism Revolution Food List on page 56.

Cauliflower Cakes

SERVES 1

INGREDIENTS	MEAL MAP A	MEAL MAP B	MEAL MAP C
CAULIFLOWER FLORETS (FROM 1 MEDIUM HEAD)	2 CUPS	4 CUPS	4 CUPS
EGGS*	2	2	2
OAT FLOUR**	¼ CUP	¼ CUP	¼ CUP
SEA SALT AND GROUND PEPPER	AS NEEDED	AS NEEDED	AS NEEDED
MIXED BERRIES	1 CUP	1 CUP	1 CUP

1. In the microwave, cook the cauliflower in a covered dish with 2 tablespoons water until soft. (Start with 3 minutes and test for softness. If it is still too firm to mash, continue to cook 1 minute at a time, testing after each minute.) Drain the cauliflower, transfer it to a bowl, and mash it with the back of a fork or a potato masher.

2. Add 1 egg, the oat flour, and salt and pepper to taste and mix. Form the mixture into patties, using about ¼ cup for each. In a large nonstick skillet, cook the patties over medium-high heat until browned on both sides, flipping them once. Transfer to a plate.

3. Beat the remaining egg in a small bowl. Pour the egg into a small nonstick skillet and cook over medium heat, stirring with a spatula to scramble the egg, until cooked to your liking.

4. Serve the cauliflower patties with the scrambled egg and berries.

*If you don't eat any animal products, you may substitute any vegetarian protein from the Metabolism Revolution Food List on page 56.

**If you don't have oat flour, pulse ½ to 1 cup of old-fashioned oats in a blender or clean coffee grinder and use what you need from this. Store the rest in the refrigerator for the next time you need oat flour.

Quinoa Scramble

SERVES 1

INGREDIENTS	MEAL MAP A	MEAL MAP B	MEAL MAP C
QUINOA	¼ CUP	¼ CUP	¼ CUP
EGGS*	2	2	4
SEA SALT AND GROUND PEPPER	DASH OF EACH	DASH OF EACH	DASH OF EACH
BABY SPINACH	2 CUPS	2 CUPS	2 CUPS
GARLIC CLOVE(S), MINCED	1	1	2
MELON	1 CUP SLICED	1 CUP SLICED	1 CUP SLICED
CUCUMBER, MEDIUM, SLICED	NONE	1	1

1. Cook the quinoa according to the package directions. Meanwhile, whisk the eggs with 1 tablespoon of water and the salt and pepper. Set aside.

2. Add the spinach and garlic to the skillet and cook for about 30 seconds. Pour the egg mixture into the skillet. Let it sit for about 10 seconds, then start pulling the eggs quickly toward the center of the pan with a wooden spoon. When the eggs look nearly cooked, add the cooked quinoa to the skillet. Mix well.

3. Transfer to a plate or bowl. Serve with the melon and, for Meal Maps B and C, the cucumber.

*If you don't eat any animal products, you may substitute any vegetarian protein from the Metabolism Revolution Food List on page 56.

Tropical Breakfast Bowl

SERVES 1

INGREDIENTS	MEAL MAP A	MEAL MAP B	MEAL MAP C
EGGS*	2	2	4
EGG WHITES*	2	2	NONE
BELL PEPPER, MUSHROOMS, ONION, BABY SPINACH, AND JALAPEÑO, IN WHATEVER PROPORTIONS YOU PREFER	2 CUPS TOTAL, CHOPPED	4 CUPS TOTAL, CHOPPED	4 CUPS TOTAL, CHOPPED
RED PEPPER FLAKES	AS NEEDED	AS NEEDED	AS NEEDED
SEA SALT AND GROUND PEPPER	AS NEEDED	AS NEEDED	AS NEEDED
BROWN RICE	½ CUP COOKED	½ CUP COOKED	½ CUP COOKED
PINEAPPLE	1 CUP DICED	1 CUP DICED	1 CUP DICED

1. In a small bowl, lightly beat the eggs (and egg whites, for Meal Maps A and B) just to combine.

2. In a large nonstick skillet, cook the vegetables over medium heat until tender. Add the egg mixture and cook, stirring with a spatula to scramble the eggs, until the eggs are cooked. Season with red pepper flakes, salt, and black pepper.

3. Serve over the brown rice. Top with the pineapple.

*If you don't eat any animal products, you may substitute any vegetarian protein from the Metabolism Revolution Food List on page 56.

Garden Hash

SERVES 1

INGREDIENTS	MEAL MAP A	MEAL MAP B	MEAL MAP C
GREEN AND/OR RED BELL PEPPER	½ CUP DICED	1 CUP DICED	1 CUP DICED
RED ONION	¼ CUP DICED	½ CUP DICED	½ CUP DICED
WATER OR BROTH	¼ CUP	¼ CUP	¼ CUP
GARLIC CLOVES, MINCED	2	3	3
FRESH ROSEMARY	1 ½ TEASPOONS	1 TABLESPOON	1 TABLESPOON
FRESH THYME	1 ½ TEASPOONS	1 TABLESPOON	1 TABLESPOON
SWEET POTATO	½ CUP CUBED	½ CUP CUBED	½ CUP CUBED
KALE	1 CUP CHOPPED LEAVES	2 CUPS CHOPPED LEAVES	2 CUPS CHOPPED LEAVES
MUSHROOMS	¼ CUP SLICED	½ CUP SLICED	½ CUP SLICED
RED PEPPER FLAKES	PINCH	PINCH	PINCH
SEA SALT AND GROUND PEPPER	AS NEEDED	AS NEEDED	AS NEEDED
EGGS*	2	2	4
PEACHES	1 CUP SLICED	1 CUP SLICED	1 CUP SLICED

1. In a medium nonstick skillet, cook the bell pepper and onion in the water or broth over medium heat. Add the garlic, rosemary, thyme, and sweet potato and cook until the sweet potato is fork-tender, about 20 minutes.

2. Add the kale, mushrooms, red pepper flakes, and salt and black pepper to taste. Cook, stirring, for about 5 minutes, until the kale wilts. Transfer the hash to a plate.

3. Cook the eggs in whatever style you like (fried, scrambled) in a non-stick skillet (don't use any oil).

4. Serve the hash with the eggs on top or to the side and the peach slices alongside.

> *If you don't eat any animal products, you may substitute any vegetarian protein from the Metabolism Revolution Food List on page 56.

Apple Slaw

SERVES 1

INGREDIENTS	MEAL MAP A	MEAL MAP B	MEAL MAP C
BEETS	1 CUP SHREDDED	2 CUPS SHREDDED	2 CUPS SHREDDED
CARROTS	1 CUP SHREDDED	2 CUPS SHREDDED	2 CUPS SHREDDED
GRANNY SMITH APPLE, CORED AND SHREDDED	1	1	1
APPLE CIDER VINEGAR	¼ CUP	½ CUP	½ CUP
SEA SALT	PINCH	PINCH	PINCH
PURE STEVIA OR BIRCH XYLITOL	AS NEEDED	AS NEEDED	AS NEEDED
BROWN RICE*	½ CUP COOKED	½ CUP COOKED	½ CUP COOKED
HARD-BOILED EGGS,** SLICED	2	2	4

1. Place the beets, carrots, and apple in a large bowl.

2. In another bowl, combine the vinegar and salt. Add the stevia or birch xylitol to taste. Pour over the veggies and apple and stir to coat. Chill for 30 minutes, if desired.

3. Serve over the brown rice with the sliced hard-boiled eggs on top.

*If you don't eat any grain, use quinoa or any other non-grain complex carb from the Metabolism Revolution Food List on page 56.

**If you don't eat any animal products, you may substitute any vegetarian protein from the Metabolism Revolution Food List on page 56.

Stuffed Pepper Breakfast

SERVES 1

INGREDIENTS	MEAL MAP A	MEAL MAP B	MEAL MAP C
BELL PEPPER(S)	1	1	2
BABY SPINACH	1 CUP CHOPPED	1 CUP CHOPPED	2 CUPS CHOPPED
TURKEY BACON,* NITRATE-FREE, COOKED AND CHOPPED	2 SLICES	4 SLICES	4 SLICES
EGG(S)*	1	2	2
SEA SALT AND GROUND PEPPER	AS NEEDED	AS NEEDED	AS NEEDED
AVOCADO, DICED	NONE	¼	¼
MIXED BERRIES	1 CUP	NONE	NONE

1. Preheat the oven to 400°F. Line a small baking dish with foil.

2. Cut off the top of the bell pepper(s) and remove the seeds. Place the pepper(s) upright in the baking dish and bake for 15 minutes.

3. Remove the pepper(s) from the oven and stuff the bottom(s) with the spinach. Add the turkey bacon. Crack the egg(s) into the pepper(s). (For Meal Map B, if both eggs don't fit in the pepper, you can cook one of the eggs separately and eat it on the side. For Meal Map C, divide all the ingredients between the two peppers.)

4. Bake for 15 to 20 minutes, or until the egg whites are set and opaque.

5. Transfer to a plate and season with salt and black pepper. For Meal Maps B and C, top with the avocado. For Meal Map A, serve with mixed berries alongside.

*If you don't eat any animal products, you may substitute any vegetarian protein from the Metabolism Revolution Food List on page 56.

Scrambled Salmon Cups

SERVES 1

INGREDIENTS	MEAL MAP A	MEAL MAP B	MEAL MAP C
EGG(S)*	1	2	2
RED ONION	¼ CUP DICED	½ CUP DICED	½ CUP DICED
SMOKED SALMON,* WILD-CAUGHT, NITRATE-FREE, NO SUGAR ADDED	2 OUNCES	4 OUNCES	4 OUNCES
SEA SALT AND GROUND PEPPER	AS NEEDED	AS NEEDED	AS NEEDED
FRESH CHIVES	GARNISH, CHOPPED	GARNISH, CHOPPED	GARNISH, CHOPPED
CUCUMBER	½ CUP THINLY SLICED	½ CUP THINLY SLICED	1 CUP THINLY SLICED
BOSTON OR BUTTER LETTUCE LEAVES	2 OR 3	2 OR 3	4 TO 6
AVOCADO, DICED	NONE	¼	¼
MELON (ANY TYPE)	1 CUP CUBED	NONE	NONE

1. In a small bowl, whisk the egg(s) well. Add a splash of water and whisk some more. Heat a medium nonstick skillet over medium heat. Add the onion and cook for 3 to 5 minutes, until soft. Add the egg(s) and use a wooden spoon or rubber spatula to gently stir the eggs until they start to firm up.

2. Add the smoked salmon to the pan and cook, stirring gently, until the eggs are completely cooked to your liking. Season with salt and pepper to taste.

3. Transfer to a plate and sprinkle the chives over the eggs. Divide the cucumber slices among the lettuce leaves and set on the plate with the eggs. For Meal Maps B and C, top the eggs with the avocado. For Meal Map A, serve with melon on the side.

*If you don't eat any animal products, you may substitute any vegetarian protein from the Metabolism Revolution Food List on page 56.

Breakfast Salad

SERVES 1

INGREDIENTS	MEAL MAP A	MEAL MAP B	MEAL MAP C
MIXED GREENS	2 CUPS	2 CUPS	4 CUPS
RED ONION	1/4 CUP DICED	1/4 CUP DICED	1/4 CUP DICED
AVOCADO, SLICED	NONE	1/4	1/4
SMOKED SALMON,* WILD-CAUGHT, NITRATE-FREE, NO SUGAR ADDED	2 OUNCES	4 OUNCES	4 OUNCES
EGG(S),* POACHED	1	2	2
SEA SALT AND GROUND PEPPER	AS NEEDED	AS NEEDED	AS NEEDED
PAPRIKA	DASH	DASH	DASH
MIXED BERRIES	1 CUP	NONE	NONE

1. On a large plate, layer the mixed greens, onion, and avocado, if following Meal Maps B and C. Place the smoked salmon around the plate.

2. Top with the poached egg(s). Season with salt and pepper to taste and sprinkle with the paprika. For Meal Map A, serve with mixed berries on the side.

*If you don't eat any animal products, you may substitute any vegetarian protein from the Metabolism Revolution Food List on page 56.

Spinach-Mushroom Frittata

SERVES 1

INGREDIENTS	MEAL MAP A	MEAL MAP B	MEAL MAP C
EGG(S)*	1	3	3
EGG WHITES*	4	NONE	NONE
WATER	¼ CUP	¼ CUP	¼ CUP
DRIED BASIL	¼ TEASPOON	¼ TEASPOON	¼ TEASPOON
DRIED OREGANO	¼ TEASPOON	¼ TEASPOON	¼ TEASPOON
DRIED THYME	¼ TEASPOON	¼ TEASPOON	¼ TEASPOON
RED PEPPER FLAKES	PINCH	PINCH	PINCH
SEA SALT AND GROUND PEPPER	AS NEEDED	AS NEEDED	AS NEEDED
TURKEY BACON,* NITRATE-FREE, CHOPPED	2 SLICES	2 SLICES	2 SLICES
GARLIC	1 TEASPOON MINCED	1 TEASPOON MINCED	1 TEASPOON MINCED
MUSHROOMS	½ CUP SLICED	½ CUP SLICED	1 CUP SLICED
WATER OR BROTH (OPTIONAL)	AS NEEDED	AS NEEDED	AS NEEDED
BABY SPINACH	1 ½ CUPS	1 ½ CUPS	3 CUPS
OLIVES, PITTED AND SLICED	NONE	8	8
APPLE	1 CUP SLICED	NONE	NONE

1. Preheat the oven to 425°F.

2. In a large bowl, whisk together the egg(s), egg whites (for Meal Map A), water, basil, oregano, thyme, red pepper flakes, and salt and black pepper to taste. Set aside.

3. Heat a large oven-safe skillet over medium-high heat. Add the bacon and cook until brown and crispy, 6 to 8 minutes. Transfer to a plate.

4. In the same skillet, cook the garlic and mushrooms, stirring occasionally and adding a little water or broth to help them cook, until tender and browned, 3 to 4 minutes.

5. Add the spinach and stir until it begins to wilt, 2 to 3 minutes. Stir in the egg mixture. Set aside 2 tablespoons of the bacon for garnish and stir in the remainder until well combined. Cook, undisturbed, until the edges of the eggs are set, about 2 minutes. Transfer the skillet to the oven and bake until the center looks set, about 8 to 10 minutes.

6. Transfer to a plate and garnish with the reserved bacon.

7. For Meal Map A, serve with apples. For Meal Maps B and C, serve with olives.

*If you don't eat any animal products, you may substitute any vegetarian protein from the Metabolism Revolution Food List on page 56.

Beefy Breakfast Skillet

SERVES 1

INGREDIENTS	MEAL MAP A	MEAL MAP B	MEAL MAP C
LEAN GROUND BEEF,* PREFERABLY GRASS-FED	2 OUNCES	4 OUNCES	4 OUNCES
ONION	¼ CUP DICED	¼ CUP DICED	½ CUP DICED
GARLIC	1 TEASPOON MINCED	1 TEASPOON MINCED	1 TEASPOON MINCED
WATER OR BROTH	2 TABLESPOONS	NONE	NONE
OLIVE OIL	NONE	1 TABLESPOON	1 TABLESPOON
KALE	2 CUPS CHOPPED LEAVES	2 CUPS CHOPPED LEAVES	4 CUPS CHOPPED LEAVES
EGG(S),* FRIED	1	2	2
SEA SALT AND GROUND PEPPER	AS NEEDED	AS NEEDED	AS NEEDED
RAW SLIVERED ALMONDS	NONE	GARNISH	GARNISH
ORANGE	1 CUP SLICED	NONE	NONE

1. Heat a nonstick skillet over medium-high heat. Add the ground beef, onion, and garlic and cook, breaking up the meat with a wooden spoon as it cooks, until browned. Remove from the heat, drain off the fat, and transfer the meat to a bowl. Set aside.

2. In the same skillet, heat the water or broth (for Meal Map A) or the olive oil (for Meal Maps B and C). Add the kale and cook until wilted. Add the ground beef and stir. Season with salt and pepper.

3. Transfer the mixture to a plate and top with the fried egg(s). For Meal Maps B and C, garnish with the slivered almonds. For Meal Map A, serve with the orange slices on the side.

*If you don't eat any animal products, you may substitute any vegetarian protein from the Metabolism Revolution Food List on page 56.

Veggie Egg Wrap

SERVES 1

INGREDIENTS	MEAL MAP A	MEAL MAP B	MEAL MAP C
BABY SPINACH	1 CUP	1 CUP	2 CUPS
MUSHROOMS	1 CUP SLICED	1 CUP SLICED	2 CUPS SLICED
ONION	2 TABLESPOONS MINCED	2 TABLESPOONS MINCED	¼ CUP MINCED
SEA SALT AND GROUND PEPPER	AS NEEDED	AS NEEDED	AS NEEDED
EGG(S)*	1	2	2
TURKEY BACON, NITRATE-FREE,* COOKED AND CRUMBLED	2 SLICES	4 SLICES	4 SLICES
OLIVES, PITTED AND SLICED	NONE	8	8
STRAWBERRIES	1 CUP SLICED	NONE	NONE

1. Heat a large nonstick skillet over medium-high heat. Add the baby spinach, mushrooms, and onion and cook, stirring, until the onion is tender and the spinach has wilted. Season with salt and pepper, remove from the heat, and set aside.

2. Heat a small nonstick skillet or omelet pan over medium-high heat. In a bowl, whisk 1 egg with a fork and pour it into the hot skillet, tilting the pan to coat the bottom with the egg. Cook for 30 seconds. Season with salt and pepper. Carefully flip the egg with a large spatula and cook for 30 seconds more, or until cooked through. Transfer the egg "wrap" to a plate. For Meal Maps B and C, repeat with the remaining egg to make a second egg "wrap."

3. Top the egg "wrap(s)" with the sautéed veggie mix, bacon, and, for Meal Map B and C, the sliced olives. For Meal Map A, serve with the strawberries on the side.

*If you don't eat any animal products, you may substitute any vegetarian protein from the Metabolism Revolution Food List on page 56.

Breakfast Bacon Collard Wrap

SERVES 1

INGREDIENTS	MEAL MAP A	MEAL MAP B	MEAL MAP C
LARGE COLLARD GREEN LEAVES	2	2	2
TURKEY BACON,* NITRATE-FREE, CHOPPED	2 SLICES	4 SLICES	4 SLICES
ONION	½ CUP DICED	½ CUP DICED	1 CUP DICED
BELL PEPPER, CUT INTO STRIPS	½	½	1
MUSHROOMS	½ CUP SLICED	½ CUP SLICED	1 CUP SLICED
SEA SALT AND GROUND PEPPER	AS NEEDED	AS NEEDED	AS NEEDED
GROUND CUMIN (OPTIONAL)	AS NEEDED	AS NEEDED	AS NEEDED
CHILI POWDER (OPTIONAL)	AS NEEDED	AS NEEDED	AS NEEDED
GARLIC POWDER (OPTIONAL)	AS NEEDED	AS NEEDED	AS NEEDED
EGG(S)*	1	2	2
AVOCADO, DICED	NONE	¼	¼
PINEAPPLE	1 CUP CUBED	NONE	NONE

1. Lay the collard green leaves facedown on a cutting board and use a sharp knife to shave down the stems so they are the same thickness as the leaves. Cut off and discard the part of the stem that extends past the leaf. Set the greens aside.

2. Heat a medium skillet over medium heat. Add the bacon and cook for about 5 minutes, until crispy, then transfer to a dish. Raise the heat to medium-high and add the onion, bell pepper, and mushrooms. Cook, stirring occasionally, until softened, 6 to 7 minutes. Season with the salt, black pepper, and, if desired, cumin, chili powder, and garlic powder. Return the bacon to the pan and stir well. Transfer to a plate and set aside. Reduce the heat under the pan to medium-low.

3. In a small bowl, whisk the egg(s) and season with salt and black pepper. Pour the egg(s) into the pan and cook, stirring with a spatula to scramble, until cooked to your liking, 3 to 4 minutes.

4. To assemble the wrap, lay a collard leaf on a plate and place half the onion–bell pepper mixture on the middle of the leaf. Layer with half the scrambled egg(s), and, for Meal Maps B and C, half the avocado. Fold the sides up to tuck, then roll like a regular tortilla. Repeat with the remaining collard leaf to make a second wrap. For Meal Map A, serve with the pineapple on the side.

*If you don't eat any animal products, you may substitute any vegetarian protein from the Metabolism Revolution Food List on page 56.

Portobello Mushroom Bake

SERVES 1

INGREDIENTS	MEAL MAP A	MEAL MAP B	MEAL MAP C
PORTOBELLO MUSHROOM CAPS	2 LARGE	2 LARGE	2 LARGE
SEA SALT	¼ TEASPOON	¼ TEASPOON	¼ TEASPOON
GROUND PEPPER	¼ TEASPOON	¼ TEASPOON	¼ TEASPOON
GARLIC POWDER	¼ TEASPOON	¼ TEASPOON	¼ TEASPOON
EGGS*	2	2	2
FRESH PARSLEY (GARNISH)	2 TABLESPOONS CHOPPED	2 TABLESPOONS CHOPPED	2 TABLESPOONS CHOPPED
AVOCADO, SLICED	NONE	¼	¼
CHERRIES	1 CUP	NONE	NONE
TURKEY BACON, NITRATE FREE,* COOKED	NONE	4 SLICES	4 SLICES

1. Preheat the broiler to high. Position a rack in the center of the oven. Line a baking sheet with aluminum foil.

2. Place the mushrooms on the prepared baking sheet and season with half the salt, half the pepper, and half the garlic powder. Place the baking sheet on the center rack and broil the mushrooms for 5 minutes on each side, or until barely tender.

3. Remove the mushrooms from the oven. Switch the oven to bake at 400°F. Turn the mushroom caps gill-side up and break an egg into each. Bake for 15 minutes, just until the whites of the eggs are cooked and opaque. Remove from the oven and sprinkle the remaining salt, pepper, and garlic powder on top.

4. Transfer the mushroom caps to a plate. Garnish with the parsley and, for Meal Maps B and C, the avocado. For Meal Map A, serve with the cherries on the side. For Meal Maps B and C, serve with the turkey bacon.

*If you don't eat any animal products, you may substitute any vegetarian protein from the Metabolism Revolution Food List on page 56.

Cauliflower "Rice" Bowl

SERVES 1

INGREDIENTS	MEAL MAP A	MEAL MAP B	MEAL MAP C
EGGS*	2	4	4
AVOCADO, SLICED	NONE	1/4	1/4
FRESH LIME JUICE	NONE	1 TEASPOON	1 TEASPOON
MUSHROOMS	1/2 CUP SLICED	1/2 CUP SLICED	1 CUP SLICED
GARLIC POWDER	AS NEEDED	AS NEEDED	AS NEEDED
CAULIFLOWER**	1 CUP RICED	1 CUP RICED	2 CUPS RICED
GARLIC CLOVES, MINCED	1	1	2
BABY SPINACH	1/2 CUP	1/2 CUP	1 CUP
GRAPEFRUIT	1 CUP SEGMENTS	NONE	NONE

1. In a small bowl, season the eggs with salt and pepper and whisk to combine. Set aside. For Meal Maps B and C, in a separate bowl, combine the avocado, lime juice, and salt and pepper to taste and mash with a fork. Set aside.

2. Heat a medium nonstick skillet over medium heat. Add the mushrooms and season with garlic powder and salt and pepper to taste, then cook, stirring, until golden brown, 5 to 8 minutes. Remove from the pan and set aside.

3. Raise the heat to medium-high, add cauliflower, and cook, stirring, for 5 minutes. Transfer the cauliflower to a bowl.

4. Return mushrooms to the skillet and reduce the heat to medium. Add minced garlic and baby spinach. Cook, stirring, for 30 seconds, or until the spinach has barely wilted, then add the eggs. Scramble with a spatula and cook to your liking. Put the egg mixture on top of the cauliflower rice.

5. For Meal Map A, serve with the grapefruit on the side. For Meal Maps B and C, top with the avocado mixture and serve.

*If you don't eat any animal products, you may substitute any vegetarian protein from the Metabolism Revolution Food List on page 56.

**To "rice" cauliflower, pulse florets in a food processor until pieces are the size of rice grains.

Broiled Cod with Nectarine Salsa Over Mixed Greens

SERVES 1

INGREDIENTS	MEAL MAP A	MEAL MAP B	MEAL MAP C
NECTARINE(S)	1	1	2
RED ONION	2 TABLESPOONS DICED	2 TABLESPOONS DICED	¼ CUP DICED
JALAPEÑO, SEEDED	1 TEASPOON FINELY CHOPPED	1 TEASPOON FINELY CHOPPED	2 TEASPOONS FINELY CHOPPED
CILANTRO, FRESH	1 TABLESPOON CHOPPED	1 TABLESPOON CHOPPED	2 TABLESPOONS CHOPPED
FRESH LIME JUICE	1 ½ TEASPOONS	1 ½ TEASPOONS	2 TABLESPOONS
SEA SALT AND GROUND PEPPER	AS NEEDED	AS NEEDED	AS NEEDED
COD FILLET*	4 OUNCES	4 OUNCES	4 OUNCES
MIXED GREENS	4 CUPS	4 CUPS	4 CUPS

1. To prepare the salsa, in a medium bowl, combine the nectarine(s), red onion, jalapeño, cilantro, lime juice, and salt and pepper to taste. Toss to combine. Cover the bowl and refrigerate for 20 to 30 minutes to allow the flavors to meld.

2. While the salsa chills, preheat the broiler. Cover a broiler pan with aluminum foil (or use a well-seasoned cast-iron skillet).

3. Season the cod with salt and pepper and set it on the prepared pan. Broil the cod until the flesh turns opaque and flakes easily, 8 to 10 minutes.

4. Serve the cod over a bed of mixed greens, topped with the salsa.

*If you don't eat any animal products, you may substitute any vegetarian protein from the Metabolism Revolution Food List on page 56.

One-Pan Tropical Chicken

SERVES 1

INGREDIENTS	MEAL MAP A	MEAL MAP B	MEAL MAP C
DRIED THYME	1 1/2 TEASPOONS	1 1/2 TEASPOONS	1 1/2 TEASPOONS
GROUND ALLSPICE	1 1/2 TEASPOONS	1 1/2 TEASPOONS	1 1/2 TEASPOONS
SEA SALT	1/4 TEASPOON	1/4 TEASPOON	1/4 TEASPOON
GROUND PEPPER	1/4 TEASPOON	1/4 TEASPOON	1/4 TEASPOON
GARLIC POWDER	3/4 TEASPOON	3/4 TEASPOON	3/4 TEASPOON
GROUND CINNAMON	1/4 TEASPOON	1/4 TEASPOON	1/4 TEASPOON
CHICKEN BREAST*	4 OUNCES	4 OUNCES	4 OUNCES
RED BELL PEPPER	1 CUP COARSELY CHOPPED	1 CUP COARSELY CHOPPED	1 CUP COARSELY CHOPPED
YELLOW BELL PEPPER	1 CUP COARSELY CHOPPED	1 CUP COARSELY CHOPPED	1 CUP COARSELY CHOPPED
RED ONION	1 CUP DICED	1 CUP DICED	1 CUP DICED
ZUCCHINI	1 CUP SMALL-DICED	1 CUP SMALL-DICED	1 CUP SMALL-DICED
MANGO CHUNKS	1 CUP	1 CUP	2 CUPS

1. Preheat the oven to 425°F. Line a baking sheet with parchment paper.

2. In a small bowl, stir together the thyme, allspice, salt, black pepper, garlic powder, and cinnamon. In a medium bowl, toss the chicken with 1 tablespoon of the spice mixture. Make sure it is evenly coated, then arrange the chicken on the prepared baking sheet. In a large bowl, toss the bell peppers, onion, and zucchini with the remaining spice mixture.

3. Bake the chicken for 10 minutes, then remove the pan from the oven and flip the chicken. Arrange the seasoned vegetables on the pan with the chicken and bake for 15 minutes more.

4. Remove from the oven and let the chicken rest for 5 minutes. Serve the chicken and veggies with the mango alongside.

*If you don't eat any animal products, you may substitute any vegetarian protein from the Metabolism Revolution Food List on page 56.

Bacon-Chicken Fruit Salad

SERVES 1

INGREDIENTS	MEAL MAP A	MEAL MAP B	MEAL MAP C
TURKEY BACON,* NITRATE-FREE	2 SLICES	2 SLICES	2 SLICES
BONELESS, SKINLESS CHICKEN BREAST*	2 OUNCES	2 OUNCES	2 OUNCES
SEA SALT	PINCH	PINCH	PINCH
GROUND PEPPER	PINCH	PINCH	PINCH
ONION POWDER	1/2 TEASPOON	1/2 TEASPOON	1/2 TEASPOON
BABY SPINACH	4 CUPS	4 CUPS	4 CUPS
MANDARIN SEGMENTS	1/2 CUP	1/2 CUP	1 CUP
STRAWBERRIES	1/2 CUP SLICED	1/2 CUP SLICED	1 CUP SLICED
BALSAMIC VINEGAR (OPTIONAL)	AS NEEDED	AS NEEDED	AS NEEDED

1. In a large deep skillet, cook the bacon over medium-high heat, stirring, until crisp, then remove from the pan and set aside.

2. Sprinkle the chicken breast with salt, pepper, and onion powder on both sides. Cook the chicken breast in the same skillet over medium heat for 2 to 4 minutes on each side, depending on the thickness of the breast. Remove from the pan and set aside to rest for 5 minutes.

3. When ready to serve, slice or chop the chicken into bite-size pieces.

4. In a large serving bowl, layer the spinach, sliced chicken, bacon, mandarin segments, and strawberries. Drizzle with balsamic vinegar, if desired, and serve.

*If you don't eat any animal products, you may substitute any vegetarian protein from the Metabolism Revolution Food List on page 56.

Pineapple-Cucumber Salad
with Sea Bass

SERVES 1

INGREDIENTS	MEAL MAP A	MEAL MAP B	MEAL MAP C
PINEAPPLE CHUNKS	1 CUP	1 CUP	2 CUPS
CUCUMBER	1 CUP SLICED	1 CUP SLICED	1 CUP SLICED
LIME, ZESTED AND JUICED	1/2	1/2	1/2
FRESH CILANTRO	2 TABLESPOONS CHOPPED	2 TABLESPOONS CHOPPED	2 TABLESPOONS CHOPPED
SEA SALT	1/2 TEASPOON, PLUS MORE AS NEEDED	1/2 TEASPOON, PLUS MORE AS NEEDED	1/2 TEASPOON, PLUS MORE AS NEEDED
GROUND PEPPER	1/2 TEASPOON, PLUS MORE AS NEEDED	1/2 TEASPOON, PLUS MORE AS NEEDED	1/2 TEASPOON, PLUS MORE AS NEEDED
SEA BASS FILLET*	4 OUNCES	4 OUNCES	4 OUNCES
PAPRIKA	1/2 TEASPOON	1/2 TEASPOON	1/2 TEASPOON
MIXED GREENS	3 CUPS	3 CUPS	3 CUPS

1. Preheat the broiler to high with the oven rack 6 to 8 inches from the heat source.

2. In a medium bowl, combine the pineapple, cucumber, lime zest, lime juice, and cilantro. Season with the salt and pepper. Toss lightly to distribute the lime zest and juice evenly. If not serving immediately, cover and refrigerate until ready to serve.

3. Season the sea bass with salt, pepper, and paprika. Place the fish on a baking sheet. Broil until the flesh is opaque and flakes easily with a fork, 10 to 12 minutes.

4. Serve the sea bass over the mixed greens, topped with the pineapple-cucumber salad.

*If you don't eat any animal products, you may substitute any vegetarian protein from the Metabolism Revolution Food List on page 56.

Turkey or Roast Beef Wraps

SERVES 1

INGREDIENTS	MEAL MAP A	MEAL MAP B	MEAL MAP C
DELI TURKEY OR ROAST BEEF,* NITRATE-FREE	4 OUNCES	4 OUNCES	4 OUNCES
CUCUMBERS, ONIONS, RADISHES, MUSHROOMS, BELL PEPPERS, ETC.	3 CUPS THINLY SLICED, TOTAL	3 CUPS THINLY SLICED, TOTAL	3 CUPS THINLY SLICED, TOTAL
LETTUCE LEAVES	4	4	4
MIXED BERRIES	1 CUP	1 CUP	2 CUPS

Wrap the deli meat and veggies in the lettuce leaves and serve with a side of the mixed berries.

*If you don't eat any animal products, you may substitute any vegetarian protein from the Metabolism Revolution Food List on page 56.

Pineapple-Ginger Chicken

SERVES 1

INGREDIENTS	MEAL MAP A	MEAL MAP B	MEAL MAP C
CHICKEN BREAST,* CUBED	4 OUNCES	4 OUNCES	4 OUNCES
SEA SALT AND GROUND PEPPER	AS NEEDED	AS NEEDED	AS NEEDED
GREEN BELL PEPPER	1 CUP 1-INCH PIECES	1 CUP 1-INCH PIECES	1 CUP 1-INCH PIECES
ONION	1 CUP 1-INCH PIECES	1 CUP 1-INCH PIECES	1 CUP 1-INCH PIECES
ASPARAGUS	2 CUPS 1-INCH PIECES	2 CUPS 1-INCH PIECES	2 CUPS 1-INCH PIECES
FRESH GINGER, PEELED	1 TABLESPOON MINCED	1 TABLESPOON MINCED	1 TABLESPOON MINCED
GARLIC	2 TEASPOONS MINCED	2 TEASPOONS MINCED	2 TEASPOONS MINCED
PINEAPPLE CHUNKS	1 CUP	1 CUP	2 CUPS
SCALLION, THINLY SLICED	GARNISH	GARNISH	GARNISH

1. Season the chicken with salt and black pepper. In a large sauté pan, cook the chicken over medium-high heat, stirring occasionally, for 5 minutes, until the chicken is cooked through and no longer pink on the inside. Transfer the chicken to a plate and set aside.

2. Add the bell pepper, onion, and asparagus to the pan. Cook, stirring occasionally, for 5 minutes, or until the veggies reach your desired level of doneness. Add the ginger, garlic, and pineapple and toss to combine. Cook, stirring, for 1 to 2 minutes more, or until the garlic is fragrant. Return the chicken to the pan and cook, stirring occasionally, for 1 to 2 minutes.

3. Transfer to a plate, garnish with sliced scallion, and serve.

*If you don't eat any animal products, you may substitute any vegetarian protein from the Metabolism Revolution Food List on page 56.

Tropical Tuna Steak

SERVES 1

INGREDIENTS	MEAL MAP A	MEAL MAP B	MEAL MAP C
MANGO	1 CUP DICED	1 CUP DICED	1 CUP DICED
RED ONION	¼ CUP DICED	¼ CUP DICED	¼ CUP DICED
RED BELL PEPPER	2 TABLESPOONS DICED	2 TABLESPOONS DICED	2 TABLESPOONS DICED
FRESH CILANTRO OR PARSLEY LEAVES	1 TABLESPOON MINCED	1 TABLESPOON MINCED	1 TABLESPOON MINCED
FRESH LIME JUICE	1 TABLESPOON	1 TABLESPOON	1 TABLESPOON
JALAPEÑO, SEEDED (OPTIONAL)	2 TEASPOONS FINELY DICED	2 TEASPOONS FINELY DICED	2 TEASPOONS FINELY DICED
SEA SALT	½ TEASPOON	½ TEASPOON	½ TEASPOON
CHILI POWDER	½ TEASPOON	½ TEASPOON	½ TEASPOON
GROUND PEPPER	GENEROUS DASH	GENEROUS DASH	GENEROUS DASH
AHI TUNA STEAK*	4 OUNCES	4 OUNCES	4 OUNCES
MIXED GREENS	4 CUPS	4 CUPS	4 CUPS
PINEAPPLE	NONE	NONE	1 CUP CUBED

1. In a medium bowl, combine the mango, onion, bell pepper, cilantro, lime juice, jalapeño, if using, and ¼ teaspoon of the salt and mix well. Set aside.

2. In a small bowl, combine the remaining ¼ teaspoon salt, the chili powder, and the black pepper. Rub this mixture on both sides of the tuna steak.

3. Preheat a nonstick skillet over medium-high heat. Add the tuna and sear for 1 to 2 minutes on each side, then remove from the heat. Let the fish rest for a couple of minutes.

4. Slice the tuna and serve the slices over the mixed greens, topped with the mango salsa. For Meal Map C, serve with the pineapple on the side.

*If you don't eat any animal products, you may substitute any vegetarian protein from the Metabolism Revolution Food List on page 56.

Very Berry Chicken Salad

SERVES 1

INGREDIENTS	MEAL MAP A	MEAL MAP B	MEAL MAP C
MIXED GREENS	2 CUPS	2 CUPS	2 CUPS
RED BELL PEPPER	1/2 CUP DICED	1/2 CUP DICED	1/2 CUP DICED
CUCUMBERS	1/2 CUP SLICED	1/2 CUP SLICED	1/2 CUP SLICED
CELERY	1/2 CUP DICED	1/2 CUP DICED	1/2 CUP DICED
ONION	1/2 CUP DICED	1/2 CUP DICED	1/2 CUP DICED
BLUEBERRIES	1/4 CUP	1/4 CUP	1/2 CUP
RASPBERRIES	1/4 CUP	1/4 CUP	1/2 CUP
STRAWBERRIES	1/4 CUP	1/4 CUP	1/2 CUP
BLACKBERRIES	1/4 CUP	1/4 CUP	1/2 CUP
GRILLED CHICKEN BREAST, CUT INTO CHUNKS*	4 OUNCES	4 OUNCES	4 OUNCES
BALSAMIC VINEGAR	2 TABLESPOONS	2 TABLESPOONS	2 TABLESPOONS
WATER	SPLASH	SPLASH	SPLASH
PURE STEVIA OR BIRCH XYLITOL	AS NEEDED	AS NEEDED	AS NEEDED

1. In a bowl, combine the mixed greens, bell pepper, cucumber, celery, onion, and berries (set aside a few berries for the dressing). Top with the grilled chicken breast.

2. In a blender, puree the reserved berries with the balsamic vinegar and a splash of water, then sweeten to taste.

3. Drizzle the dressing over the salad, toss, and serve with the stevia.

*If you don't eat any animal products, you may substitute any vegetarian protein from the Metabolism Revolution Food List on page 56.

Stuffed Acorn Squash

SERVES 1

INGREDIENTS	MEAL MAP A	MEAL MAP B	MEAL MAP C
ACORN SQUASH, SEEDED	1/2	1/2	1/2
GARLIC	1/2 TEASPOON MINCED	1/2 TEASPOON MINCED	1/2 TEASPOON MINCED
ONION	1/2 CUP DICED	1/2 CUP DICED	1/2 CUP DICED
WATER	SPLASH	SPLASH	SPLASH
LEAN GROUND TURKEY*	4 OUNCES	4 OUNCES	4 OUNCES
APPLE	1 CUP DICED	1 CUP DICED	2 CUPS DICED
FRESH ROSEMARY	3/4 TEASPOON	3/4 TEASPOON	3/4 TEASPOON
FRESH THYME	1 1/2 TEASPOONS	1 1/2 TEASPOONS	1 1/2 TEASPOONS
BABY SPINACH	2 CUPS	2 CUPS	2 CUPS

1. Preheat oven to 400°F. Line a baking sheet with parchment paper.

2. Place the squash cut-side down on the baking sheet and roast for 20 to 30 minutes, or until the top of the squash feels tender when gently pressed. Remove from the oven and set aside.

3. While the squash roasts, heat a large saucepan over medium-low heat. Add garlic and onion with a splash of water and cook until just tender, about 6 minutes. Add turkey, increase heat to medium, and cook for 5 to 8 minutes until just browned. Add the apple, rosemary, and thyme and cook, stirring, until the apple softens. Add the spinach and salt and pepper to taste and cook, stirring, until the spinach wilts.

4. Preheat the broiler. While broiler preheats, fill the squash cavities with the stuffing mixture. Arrange the squash on the baking sheet, stuffing-side up, and broil for 5 to 10 minutes, until the top gets nice and toasty. Once browned, remove from the oven, allow to cool a bit, and serve warm.

*If you don't eat any animal products, you may substitute any vegetarian protein from the Metabolism Revolution Food List on page 56.

LUNCHES, PART 2

Shrimp Salad

SERVES 1

INGREDIENTS	MEAL MAP A	MEAL MAP B	MEAL MAP C
SHRIMP,* FRESH OR DEFROSTED, PEELED (ANY SIZE)	4 OUNCES	4 OUNCES	8 OUNCES
SAFFLOWER OIL MAYONNAISE**	¼ CUP	¼ CUP	¼ CUP
FRESH LEMON JUICE	½ TEASPOON	½ TEASPOON	½ TEASPOON
DRIED DILL	¼ TEASPOON	¼ TEASPOON	¼ TEASPOON
OLD BAY SEASONING	¼ TEASPOON	¼ TEASPOON	¼ TEASPOON
RED ONION	2 TABLESPOONS DICED	2 TABLESPOONS DICED	2 TABLESPOONS DICED
CELERY	¼ CUP DICED	¼ CUP DICED	¼ CUP DICED
SPRING GREENS	2 CUPS	4 CUPS	4 CUPS

1. In a medium saucepan, bring 1 ½ cups water to a simmer over medium heat. Add the shrimp and cook for 2 to 3 minutes, or until pink and just cooked through (do not overcook). Drain the shrimp in a colander, rinse with cold water, and allow to cool.

2. While the shrimp are cooling, in a medium bowl, whisk together the mayonnaise, lemon juice, dill, and Old Bay Seasoning. Cover and refrigerate until ready to use.

3. Peel and devein the shrimp and cut them in half (or chop them, if you prefer). Add the shrimp, onion, and celery to the bowl with the mayonnaise mixture and stir well to coat. Cover and refrigerate for at least 1 hour before serving.

4. Serve over the greens.

*If you don't eat any animal products, you may substitute any vegetarian protein from the Metabolism Revolution Food List on page 56.

**If you don't eat eggs, you can use olive oil or any other oil on the food list in place of safflower oil mayonnaise.

Tuna-Stuffed Avocado

SERVES 1

INGREDIENTS	MEAL MAP A	MEAL MAP B	MEAL MAP C
AVOCADO, SMALL	1/2	1/2	1/2
CANNED TUNA* IN WATER, DRAINED	4 OUNCES	4 OUNCES	8 OUNCES
RED BELL PEPPER	1/4 CUP DICED	1/4 CUP DICED	1/2 CUP DICED
JALAPEÑO, SEEDED	1 TABLESPOON MINCED	1 TABLESPOON MINCED	2 TABLESPOONS MINCED
FRESH CILANTRO LEAVES	1/4 CUP CHOPPED	1/4 CUP CHOPPED	1/2 CUP CHOPPED
FRESH LIME JUICE	1 TABLESPOON	1 TABLESPOON	2 TABLESPOONS
SEA SALT AND GROUND PEPPER	AS NEEDED	AS NEEDED	AS NEEDED
CUCUMBER	1/2 CUP SLICED	1 CUP SLICED	1 CUP SLICED
CELERY, CUT INTO STICKS	3 STALKS	4 STALKS	4 STALKS
CARROT, CUT INTO STICKS	NONE	1 CUP	1 CUP

1. Scoop out some of the avocado from the pitted area to widen the "bowl." Set the half aside. Place the scooped avocado in a medium bowl and mash it with a fork.

2. Add the tuna, bell pepper, jalapeño, cilantro, and lime juice and stir until well combined.

3. Scoop the tuna mixture into the avocado half. Season with salt and black pepper. Serve with the sliced cucumber, celery sticks, and, for Meal Maps B and C, carrot sticks.

*If you don't eat any animal products, you may substitute any vegetarian protein from the Metabolism Revolution Food List on page 56.

Lemon Shrimp Bowl

SERVES 1

INGREDIENTS	MEAL MAP A	MEAL MAP B	MEAL MAP C
ZUCCHINI NOODLES*	2 CUPS	2 CUPS	2 CUPS
LEMON HUMMUS**	¼ CUP	¼ CUP	¼ CUP
COOKED SHRIMP***	4 OUNCES	4 OUNCES	8 OUNCES
SEA SALT AND GROUND PEPPER	AS NEEDED	AS NEEDED	AS NEEDED
CUCUMBER	NONE	1 CUP SLICED	1 CUP SLICED
CARROT STICKS	NONE	1 CUP	1 CUP

1. In a large skillet, heat the zucchini noodles over medium-high heat. Add the hummus and shrimp. Cook, stirring, until the entire dish is hot and well mixed, about 5 minutes. (It will take some time for the hummus to melt and cover the zoodles.) Season with salt and pepper.

2. Remove from the heat and serve. For Meal Maps B and C, serve with the cucumber and carrot sticks on the side.

*Turn your zucchini into long noodles using a spiralizer, food processor slicing blade, vegetable peeler, or just a sharp knife.

**If you can't find lemon hummus, use regular hummus and add 2 tablespoons fresh lemon juice and ½ teaspoon ground pepper.

***If you don't eat any animal products, you may substitute any vegetarian protein from the Metabolism Revolution Food List on page 56.

Asparagus and Bacon Salad

SERVES 1

INGREDIENTS	MEAL MAP A	MEAL MAP B	MEAL MAP C
ASPARAGUS	2 CUPS CUT INTO 1-INCH PIECES	4 CUPS CUT INTO 1-INCH PIECES	4 CUPS CUT INTO 1-INCH PIECES
OLIVE OIL	¼ CUP	¼ CUP	¼ CUP
APPLE CIDER VINEGAR	¼ CUP	¼ CUP	¼ CUP
GARLIC	½ TEASPOON MINCED	½ TEASPOON MINCED	½ TEASPOON MINCED
BIRCH XYLITOL (OPTIONAL, IF YOU LIKE A SWEETER DRESSING)	1 ½ TEASPOONS	1 ½ TEASPOONS	1 ½ TEASPOONS
SEA SALT AND GROUND PEPPER	AS NEEDED	AS NEEDED	AS NEEDED
HARD-BOILED EGG(S),* SLICED	1	1	2
TURKEY BACON,* NITRATE-FREE, COOKED AND CRUMBLED	2 SLICES	2 SLICES	4 SLICES

1. Bring a pot of water to a boil, add the asparagus, and cook for 2 to 3 minutes, until tender yet firm. Drain and run under cold water to stop the cooking. Chop and set aside.

2. In a small bowl, mix the oil, vinegar, garlic, and birch xylitol, if using. Season with salt and pepper.

3. Arrange the asparagus on a plate, top with the egg(s) and bacon, and drizzle with the vinaigrette. Serve.

*If you don't eat any animal products, you may substitute any vegetarian protein from the Metabolism Revolution Food List on page 56.

Mexican Fiesta Chicken Salad

SERVES 1

INGREDIENTS	MEAL MAP A	MEAL MAP B	MEAL MAP C
FRESH LIME JUICE	2 TEASPOONS	2 TEASPOONS	2 TEASPOONS
PURE STEVIA	1/2 TEASPOON	1/2 TEASPOON	1/2 TEASPOON
OLIVE OIL	1 TABLESPOON	1 TABLESPOON	1 TABLESPOON
GARLIC	1/2 TEASPOON MINCED	1/2 TEASPOON MINCED	1/2 TEASPOON MINCED
BONELESS, SKINLESS CHICKEN BREAST*	4 OUNCES	4 OUNCES	8 OUNCES
GROUND CHIPOTLE	1/8 TEASPOON	1/8 TEASPOON	1/8 TEASPOON
DRIED OREGANO	1/8 TEASPOON	1/8 TEASPOON	1/8 TEASPOON
GROUND CUMIN	1/8 TEASPOON	1/8 TEASPOON	1/8 TEASPOON
MIXED GREENS	1 1/2 CUPS	3 CUPS	3 CUPS
FRESH CILANTRO LEAVES	1 1/2 TEASPOONS CHOPPED	1 TABLESPOON CHOPPED	1 TABLESPOON CHOPPED
AVOCADO, SMALL, DICED	1/4	1/4	1/4
CUCUMBER	1/4 CUP SLICED	1/4 CUP SLICED	1/4 CUP SLICED
RED BELL PEPPER	1/4 CUP DICED	1/4 CUP DICED	1/4 CUP DICED
RED ONION	1/4 CUP DICED	1/2 CUP DICED	1/2 CUP DICED
LIME, CUT INTO WEDGES	1/8	1/8	1/8

1. In a jar, combine lime juice, stevia, oil, garlic, and salt and black pepper to taste. Seal and shake well.

2. Slice the chicken and season with chipotle, oregano, cumin, 1/8 teaspoon salt, and 1/8 teaspoon black pepper. Cook in a medium skillet over medium-low heat for 8 minutes, or until cooked through.

3. Place the mixed greens and cilantro in a bowl. Top with avocado, cucumber, bell pepper, onion, and chicken. Drizzle with salad dressing, garnish with lime wedges, and serve.

*If you don't eat any animal products, you may substitute any vegetarian protein from the Metabolism Revolution Food List on page 56.

Tuna-Avocado Salad

SERVES 1

INGREDIENTS	MEAL MAP A	MEAL MAP B	MEAL MAP C
CANNED TUNA* IN WATER, DRAINED AND FLAKED	4 OUNCES	4 OUNCES	8 OUNCES
CUCUMBER	½ CUP DICED	1 CUP DICED	1 CUP DICED
AVOCADO, DICED	¼	¼	¼
RED ONION	¼ CUP DICED	¼ CUP DICED	¼ CUP DICED
FRESH CILANTRO LEAVES	1 ½ TEASPOONS CHOPPED	1 TABLESPOON CHOPPED	1 TABLESPOON CHOPPED
OLIVE OIL	1 TEASPOON	2 TEASPOONS	2 TEASPOONS
FRESH LEMON JUICE	1 TEASPOON	2 TEASPOONS	2 TEASPOONS
SEA SALT AND GROUND PEPPER	AS NEEDED	AS NEEDED	AS NEEDED
MIXED GREENS	1 ½ CUPS	3 CUPS	3 CUPS

1. In a large salad bowl, combine the tuna, cucumber, avocado, onion, and cilantro.

2. Drizzle the salad with the oil and lemon juice and season it with salt and pepper. Toss to combine and serve over the mixed greens.

*If you don't eat any animal products, you may substitute any vegetarian protein from the Metabolism Revolution Food List on page 56.

Shredded Chicken and Green Bean Salad

SERVES 1

INGREDIENTS	MEAL MAP A	MEAL MAP B	MEAL MAP C
JALAPEÑO, SEEDED AND DICED	1	2	2
LIMES, JUICED	1 ½	3	3
GARLIC	½ TEASPOON MINCED	1 TEASPOON MINCED	1 TEASPOON MINCED
GROUND ALLSPICE	1 ½ TEASPOONS	1 TABLESPOON	1 TABLESPOON
DRIED THYME	½ TEASPOON	1 TEASPOON	1 TEASPOON
BIRCH XYLITOL	¾ TEASPOON	1 ½ TEASPOONS	1 ½ TEASPOONS
OLIVE OIL	1 ½ TEASPOONS	1 TABLESPOON	1 TABLESPOON
CHICKEN,* COOKED AND SHREDDED	4 OUNCES	4 OUNCES	8 OUNCES
GREEN BEANS, COOKED	2 CUPS	4 CUPS	4 CUPS
UNSWEETENED SHREDDED COCONUT	⅛ CUP	⅛ CUP	⅛ CUP
SEA SALT AND GROUND PEPPER	AS NEEDED	AS NEEDED	AS NEEDED

1. In a small bowl, combine the jalapeño, lime juice, garlic, allspice, thyme, birch xylitol, and oil and stir to combine.

2. In a serving bowl, combine the shredded chicken, green beans, and coconut. Pour in the dressing and toss to combine. Season with salt and pepper and serve.

*If you don't eat any animal products, you may substitute any vegetarian protein from the Metabolism Revolution Food List on page 56.

Fajita Chicken Bowl

SERVES 1

INGREDIENTS	MEAL MAP A	MEAL MAP B	MEAL MAP C
OLIVE OIL	1 1/2 TEASPOONS	1 1/2 TEASPOONS	1 TABLESPOON
FRESH LIME JUICE	1 TABLESPOON	1 TABLESPOON	1 TABLESPOON
GARLIC	1/2 TEASPOON MINCED	1/2 TEASPOON MINCED	1 TEASPOON MINCED
SMOKED OR REGULAR PAPRIKA	1/4 TEASPOON	1/4 TEASPOON	1/2 TEASPOON
SEA SALT	1/4 TEASPOON	1/4 TEASPOON	1/2 TEASPOON
RED PEPPER FLAKES	PINCH	PINCH	PINCH
CHICKEN BREAST,* CUT INTO STRIPS	4 OUNCES	4 OUNCES	8 OUNCES
BELL PEPPER	1 CUP	1 1/2 CUPS	2 CUPS
WHITE ONION	1/2 CUP SLICED (HALF-MOONS)	1/2 CUP SLICED (HALF-MOONS)	1 CUP SLICED (HALF-MOONS)
MIXED GREENS	1 CUP	2 CUPS	2 CUPS
AVOCADO, DICED	1/4	1/4	1/4

1. In a small bowl, whisk together the oil, lime juice, garlic, paprika, salt, and red pepper flakes. Put the chicken strips into a zip-top freezer bag. Pour the marinade over the chicken, seal the bag, and shake to coat. Marinate in the refrigerator for at least 1 hour or up to overnight.

2. Heat a large nonstick skillet over medium-high heat. Drain the chicken and discard the marinade. Put the chicken, bell pepper, and onion in the pan and cook until the vegetables are crisp-tender and the chicken is cooked through, about 8 minutes.

3. Serve over the mixed greens, topped with the avocado.

*If you don't eat any animal products, you may substitute any vegetarian protein from the Metabolism Revolution Food List on page 56.

Kale Skillet

SERVES 1

INGREDIENTS	MEAL MAP A	MEAL MAP B	MEAL MAP C
OLIVE OIL	1 TABLESPOON	1 TABLESPOON	1 TABLESPOON
GARLIC	1 TEASPOON MINCED	2 TEASPOONS MINCED	2 TEASPOONS MINCED
ONION	1/4 CUP MINCED	1/2 CUP MINCED	1/2 CUP MINCED
KALE, STEMMED, LEAVES CHOPPED	2 1/2 OUNCES	4 1/2 OUNCES	4 1/2 OUNCES
EGGS*	2	4	4
SLICED RAW ALMONDS	2 TABLESPOONS	2 TABLESPOONS	2 TABLESPOONS

1. In a medium nonstick skillet, heat the oil over medium heat. Add the garlic and onion. Cook, stirring, until the onion is translucent.

2. Add the kale and cook until slightly wilted. In a small bowl, whisk the eggs and add to the kale mixture. Cook, stirring with a spatula to scramble, until cooked to your liking.

3. Garnish with the sliced almonds and serve.

*If you don't eat any animal products, you may substitute any vegetarian protein from the Metabolism Revolution Food List on page 56.

Spicy Tips

SERVES 1

INGREDIENTS	MEAL MAP A	MEAL MAP B	MEAL MAP C
OLIVE OIL	1 TABLESPOON	1 TABLESPOON	1 TABLESPOON
SMOKED PAPRIKA	1/4 TEASPOON	1/4 TEASPOON	1/4 TEASPOON
GARLIC	1/4 TEASPOON MINCED	1/4 TEASPOON MINCED	1/4 TEASPOON MINCED
CAYENNE PEPPER	DASH	DASH	DASH
SEA SALT AND GROUND PEPPER	AS NEEDED	AS NEEDED	AS NEEDED
STEAK OF CHOICE,* CUT INTO 2-INCH PIECES	4 OUNCES	4 OUNCES	8 OUNCES
ASPARAGUS	1 CUP 1-INCH PIECES	2 CUPS 1-INCH PIECES	2 CUPS 1-INCH PIECES
BROCCOLI FLORETS	1 CUP	2 CUPS	2 CUPS

1. In a large zip-top freezer bag, combine the oil, paprika, garlic, cayenne, and salt and black pepper to taste. Add the steak, seal, and shake the bag to coat the meat fully. Set aside to marinate for 30 minutes to 2 hours.

2. Meanwhile, fill a large pot with 1 inch of water and set a steamer basket inside. Bring the water to a simmer. Add the asparagus and broccoli to the steamer basket, cover, and steam until crisp-tender.

3. Preheat the broiler.

4. Drain the steak and discard the marinade. Place the steak onto a large baking sheet and broil for 4 to 8 minutes, or until cooked to the desired doneness.

5. Serve the steak with the steamed asparagus and broccoli florets.

*If you don't eat any animal products, you may substitute any vegetarian protein from the Metabolism Revolution Food List on page 56.

DINNERS, PART 1

Steak, Mushroom, and Sweet Potato Kebabs

SERVES 1

INGREDIENTS	MEAL MAP A	MEAL MAP B	MEAL MAP C
STEAK,* CUT INTO 1-INCH CHUNKS	4 OUNCES	4 OUNCES	8 OUNCES
MUSHROOMS, STEMMED	4 OUNCES	8 OUNCES	8 OUNCES
BALSAMIC VINEGAR	1/8 CUP	1/8 CUP	1/4 CUP
SEA SALT	1/8 TEASPOON	1/8 TEASPOON	1/8 TEASPOON
GROUND PEPPER	1/8 TEASPOON	1/8 TEASPOON	1/4 TEASPOON
FRESH ROSEMARY	1/8 TEASPOON	1/8 TEASPOON	1/4 TEASPOON
DRIED OREGANO	1/8 TEASPOON	1/8 TEASPOON	1/4 TEASPOON
GARLIC	1 TEASPOON MINCED	1 TEASPOON MINCED	2 TEASPOONS MINCED
SWEET POTATO, LARGE, CUT INTO 2-INCH CUBES	1/2	1/2	1/2
GREEN BEANS	1 CUP	2 CUPS	2 CUPS
RED ONION	1/2 CUP BITE-SIZE CHUNKS	1 CUP BITE-SIZE CHUNKS	1 CUP BITE-SIZE CHUNKS

1. If using wooden or bamboo skewers, soak them in water for 30 minutes before using to avoid burning.

2. Arrange the steak and mushrooms in an even layer on a rimmed baking sheet.

3. In a medium bowl, whisk together the vinegar, salt, pepper, rosemary, oregano, and garlic. Pour the mixture over the steak and mushrooms. Cover and refrigerate for at least 2 hours.

4. Meanwhile, bring a large pot of salted water to a boil. Add the sweet potato and boil until just tender, 8 to 10 minutes. Drain and let cool slightly. You could set the green beans in a steamer basket over the

boiling water and cook two things at once, or steam them separately in a steamer. Either way, steam the beans for 3 to 5 minutes, or until crisp-tender and bright green.

5. When ready to cook, heat a grill to medium-high or heat a grill pan over medium-high heat.

6. Thread the steak, mushrooms, sweet potato, and onion onto the skewers. Grill the kebabs for 10 to 12 minutes, turning once, until the meat is cooked to the desired doneness.

7. Season with salt and pepper and serve with the green beans.

*If you don't eat any animal products, you may substitute any vegetarian protein from the Metabolism Revolution Food List on page 56.

Lemon-Basil Pork Chops
with Wild Rice

SERVES 1

INGREDIENTS	MEAL MAP A	MEAL MAP B	MEAL MAP C
FRESH BASIL	1/4 CUP MINCED	1/4 CUP MINCED	1/2 CUP MINCED
GARLIC	2 1/4 TEASPOONS MINCED	2 1/4 TEASPOONS MINCED	1 TABLESPOON PLUS 1 TEASPOON, MINCED
FRESH LEMON JUICE	2 1/4 TEASPOONS, PLUS MORE AS NEEDED	2 1/4 TEASPOONS	1 TABLESPOON PLUS 1 TEASPOON
SEA SALT	1/4 TEASPOON, PLUS MORE AS NEEDED	1/4 TEASPOON, PLUS MORE AS NEEDED	1/2 TEASPOON, PLUS MORE AS NEEDED
GROUND PEPPER	1/8 TEASPOON, PLUS MORE AS NEEDED	1/8 TEASPOON, PLUS MORE AS NEEDED	1/4 TEASPOON, PLUS MORE AS NEEDED
PORK LOIN CHOP,* THICK-CUT	4 OUNCES	4 OUNCES	8 OUNCES
WILD RICE	1/2 CUP COOKED	1/2 CUP COOKED	1/2 CUP COOKED
ASPARAGUS	2 CUPS 1-INCH PIECES	4 CUPS 1-INCH PIECES	4 CUPS 1-INCH PIECES

1. In a small bowl, combine the basil, garlic, lemon juice, salt, and pepper and mix well.

2. Coat both sides of the pork chop with the mixture and let sit for 20 minutes. Steam the asparagus in a steamer or steamer basket over boiling water for about 5 minutes, or until crisp-tender and bright green.

3. Heat a grill to medium or heat a grill pan over medium heat.

4. Grill the chop over direct heat for 5 to 6 minutes per side, or until the internal temperature reaches 145°F. Let rest for 5 minutes.

5. Season the chop with the salt and pepper and drizzle with additional lemon juice. Serve with the wild rice and steamed asparagus alongside.

*If you don't eat any animal products, you may substitute any vegetarian protein from the Metabolism Revolution Food List on page 56.

Steak and Quinoa Bowl

SERVES 1

INGREDIENTS	MEAL MAP A	MEAL MAP B	MEAL MAP C
ANGUS STEAK*	4 OUNCES	4 OUNCES	8 OUNCES
GARLIC POWDER	¼ TEASPOON	¼ TEASPOON	¼ TEASPOON
SEA SALT AND GROUND PEPPER	AS NEEDED	AS NEEDED	AS NEEDED
QUINOA	½ CUP COOKED	½ CUP COOKED	½ CUP COOKED
CUCUMBER	1 CUP SLICED	2 CUPS SLICED	2 CUPS SLICED
RED BELL PEPPER	1 CUP COARSELY CHOPPED	2 CUPS COARSELY CHOPPED	2 CUPS COARSELY CHOPPED
FRESH BASIL LEAVES, CHOPPED	3	5	5
SCALLIONS	1 TABLESPOON DICED	2 TABLESPOONS DICED	2 TABLESPOONS DICED
BALSAMIC VINEGAR (OPTIONAL)	AS NEEDED	AS NEEDED	AS NEEDED

1. Heat a grill to medium or heat a grill pan over medium-high heat.

2. Season the steak with the garlic powder, salt, and black pepper. Grill for about 3 minutes on each side for medium-rare (although the time will depend on the thickness of your steak). Remove the steak from the grill and let rest for 5 minutes, then slice thinly.

3. Place the quinoa in a bowl and top with the steak. Add the cucumber, bell pepper, basil, and scallions, drizzle the vegetables with vinegar, if using, and season with salt and black pepper. Serve.

*If you don't eat any animal products, you may substitute any vegetarian protein from the Metabolism Revolution Food List on page 56.

Cajun Shrimp and Black Beans

SERVES 1

INGREDIENTS	MEAL MAP A	MEAL MAP B	MEAL MAP C
CAJUN SEASONING	1/4 TEASPOON	1/4 TEASPOON	1/2 TEASPOON
GROUND PEPPER	1/8 TEASPOON, PLUS MORE AS NEEDED	1/8 TEASPOON, PLUS MORE AS NEEDED	1/2 TEASPOON, PLUS MORE AS NEEDED
CHILI POWDER	3/4 TEASPOON	3/4 TEASPOON	1 1/4 TEASPOONS
ONION POWDER	3/4 TEASPOON	3/4 TEASPOON	1 1/4 TEASPOONS
GROUND CUMIN	1/4 TEASPOON	1/4 TEASPOON	1/2 TEASPOON
SMOKED PAPRIKA	3/4 TEASPOON	3/4 TEASPOON	1 1/2 TEASPOONS
RAW SHRIMP,* MEDIUM SIZE, PEELED AND DEVEINED, FRESH OR DEFROSTED	4 OUNCES	4 OUNCES	8 OUNCES
LIME, JUICED	1/2	1/2	1/2
FRESH CILANTRO, CHOPPED	AS NEEDED	AS NEEDED	AS NEEDED
BLACK BEANS, CANNED (OR DRIED BLACK BEANS YOU HAVE ALREADY SOAKED AND COOKED)	1/2 CUP DRAINED AND RINSED	1/2 CUP DRAINED AND RINSED	1/2 CUP DRAINED AND RINSED
CAULIFLOWER FLORETS	2 CUPS	4 CUPS	4 CUPS

1. Preheat the oven to 450°F. Line a baking sheet with aluminum foil.

2. In a large bowl, combine the Cajun seasoning, pepper, chili powder, onion powder, cumin, and paprika and mix well. Add the shrimp and coat evenly.

3. Spread the seasoned shrimp in an even layer on the prepared baking sheet. Bake for 10 to 12 minutes. Remove from the oven, squeeze the lime juice over the entire pan, and sprinkle with cilantro and salt and pepper as needed.

4. While the shrimp is cooking, steam the cauliflower florets in a steamer or in a steamer basket over boiling water for about 5 minutes, or until crisp-tender.

5. Serve the shrimp with the warmed black beans and cauliflower florets.

*If you don't eat any animal products, you may substitute any vegetarian protein from the Metabolism Revolution Food List on page 56.

Chicken and Black Bean–Stuffed Pepper Tacos

SERVES 1

INGREDIENTS	MEAL MAP A	MEAL MAP B	MEAL MAP C
BONELESS, SKINLESS CHICKEN BREAST*	4 OUNCES	4 OUNCES	8 OUNCES
GARLIC POWDER	1/4 TEASPOON	1/4 TEASPOON	1/4 TEASPOON
DRIED OREGANO	1/4 TEASPOON	1/4 TEASPOON	1/4 TEASPOON
CHILI POWDER	1 1/8 TEASPOONS	1 1/8 TEASPOONS	1 1/8 TEASPOONS
GROUND CUMIN	1 TEASPOON	1 TEASPOON	1 TEASPOON
BLACK BEANS, CANNED	1/2 CUP DRAINED AND RINSED	1/2 CUP DRAINED AND RINSED	1/2 CUP DRAINED AND RINSED
WHITE ONION	1 CUP THINLY SLICED	1 CUP THINLY SLICED	1 CUP THINLY SLICED
GREEN CHILES	1 (4-OUNCE) CAN	1 (4-OUNCE) CAN	1 (4-OUNCE) CAN
WATER (OPTIONAL)	1/4 TO 1/2 CUP	1/4 TO 1/2 CUP	1/4 TO 1/2 CUP
BELL PEPPER	1	1	1
CABBAGE	1 CUP SHREDDED	2 CUPS SHREDDED	2 CUPS SHREDDED
FRESH CILANTRO LEAVES	1 1/2 TEASPOONS MINCED	1 TABLESPOON MINCED	1 TABLESPOON MINCED
FRESH LIME JUICE	1 TEASPOON	2 TEASPOONS	2 TEASPOONS
SEA SALT AND GROUND PEPPER	AS NEEDED	AS NEEDED	AS NEEDED
FRESH CILANTRO OR PARSLEY, CHOPPED	GARNISH	GARNISH	GARNISH

1. Preheat the oven to 375°F.

2. Put the chicken breast in a small baking dish with a lid (or use aluminum foil). Add the garlic powder, oregano, chili powder, and cumin and toss to coat. Add the black beans, onion, and green chiles. If the mixture seems dry, add the water. Cover the baking dish and put it in the oven. Bake until the chicken is cooked through and the mixture is fully heated, about 15 minutes for Meal Maps A and B, or about 25 minutes for Meal Map C. Remove from the oven and shred the chicken, mixing it in with the beans and vegetables.

3. Remove the top from the bell pepper and halve the pepper lengthwise to make two "boats."

4. In a medium bowl, mix the cabbage, cilantro, lime juice, and as much salt and pepper as you like. Stuff the pepper halves with 1 cup of the cabbage mixture and ½ cup of the chicken-bean mixture.

5. Garnish with cilantro and serve. (You can pick these up with your hands and eat them just like tacos.)

*If you don't eat any animal products, you may substitute any vegetarian protein from the Metabolism Revolution Food List on page 56.

Steak and Cabbage Sauté with Sweet Potato Mash

SERVES 1

INGREDIENTS	MEAL MAP A	MEAL MAP B	MEAL MAP C
STEAK*	4 OUNCES	4 OUNCES	8 OUNCES
SEA SALT AND GROUND PEPPER	AS NEEDED	AS NEEDED	AS NEEDED
GARLIC	1 TEASPOON MINCED	1 TEASPOON MINCED	1 TEASPOON MINCED
ONION	½ CUP CHOPPED	½ CUP CHOPPED	½ CUP CHOPPED
CABBAGE	1 CUP CHOPPED	2 CUPS CHOPPED	2 CUPS CHOPPED
FRESH GREEN BEANS	1 CUP	1 ½ CUPS	1 ½ CUPS
SWEET POTATO, LARGE, BAKED	½	½	½
GARLIC POWDER	PINCH	PINCH	PINCH
THYME, FRESH OR DRIED	PINCH	PINCH	PINCH

1. Heat a grill to medium-high or heat a grill pan over medium-high heat.

2. Season the steak with salt and pepper and grill until cooked to your desired doneness.

3. Let rest for a few minutes, then slice and set aside.

4. In a medium nonstick skillet, cook the garlic and onion over medium heat, stirring, until tender. Add the cabbage and cook until the cabbage is crisp-tender, about 6 minutes. Stir in the steak.

5. Steam the green beans in a steamer or over boiling water until crisp-tender and bright green, about 6 minutes.

6. In a bowl, mash the sweet potato and season with the garlic powder, thyme, salt, and pepper. Top with the steak and cabbage. Serve with the green beans on the side.

*If you don't eat any animal products, you may substitute any vegetarian protein from the Metabolism Revolution Food List on page 56.

Mexican Zucchini Bowl

SERVES 1

INGREDIENTS	MEAL MAP A	MEAL MAP B	MEAL MAP C
LEAN GROUND BEEF*	4 OUNCES	4 OUNCES	8 OUNCES
RED BELL PEPPER	1 CUP DICED	1 CUP DICED	1 CUP DICED
RED ONION	2 TABLESPOONS MINCED	2 TABLESPOONS MINCED	1/4 CUP MINCED
MUSHROOMS	1/2 CUP SLICED	1/2 CUP SLICED	1/2 CUP SLICED
GARLIC	2 TEASPOONS MINCED	2 1/2 TEASPOONS MINCED	4 TEASPOONS MINCED
SEA SALT	1 TEASPOON	1 1/2 TEASPOONS	2 TEASPOONS
GROUND PEPPER	1/2 TEASPOON	3/4 TEASPOON	1 TEASPOON
CHILI POWDER	1 TABLESPOON	1 1/2 TABLESPOONS	2 TABLESPOONS
RED PEPPER FLAKES (OPTIONAL)	1/4 TEASPOON	1/4 TEASPOON	1/2 TEASPOON
GROUND CUMIN	1 TEASPOON	1 1/2 TEASPOONS	2 TEASPOONS
BLACK BEANS, CANNED (OR DRIED THAT YOU HAVE ALREADY SOAKED AND COOKED)	1/2 CUP DRAINED AND RINSED	1/2 CUP DRAINED AND RINSED	1/2 CUP DRAINED AND RINSED
ZUCCHINI	1 CUP DICED	1 CUP DICED	1 CUP DICED

In a large nonstick skillet, combine the ground beef, bell pepper, onion, mushrooms, garlic, salt, and black pepper and cook over medium heat until the meat is lightly browned. Add the chili powder, red pepper flakes, if using, cumin, black beans, and zucchini. Cover and cook for about 10 minutes, until the zucchini is cooked through but still firm. Serve.

*If you don't eat any animal products, you may substitute any vegetarian protein from the Metabolism Revolution Food List on page 56.

Sweet Potato–Shrimp Cooked Salad

SERVES 1

INGREDIENTS	MEAL MAP A	MEAL MAP B	MEAL MAP C
YELLOW ONION	1/4 CUP THINLY SLICED	1/2 CUP THINLY SLICED	1/2 CUP THINLY SLICED
GARLIC	1 TEASPOON MINCED	2 TEASPOONS MINCED	2 TEASPOONS MINCED
GROUND CUMIN	1/2 TEASPOON	1/2 TEASPOON	1/2 TEASPOON
SWEET POTATO	1/2 CUP CUBED	1/2 CUP CUBED	1/2 CUP CUBED
SHRIMP,* RAW, FRESH OR DEFROSTED, PEELED (ANY SIZE)	4 OUNCES	4 OUNCES	8 OUNCES
BABY KALE OR SPINACH	2 CUPS	3 1/2 CUPS	3 1/2 CUPS
SEA SALT AND GROUND PEPPER	AS NEEDED	AS NEEDED	AS NEEDED

1. In a medium nonstick skillet, add the onion. Cook over medium heat until it is softened and golden, about 8 minutes.

2. Add the garlic and cumin and cook for about 30 seconds. Add the sweet potato and cook until fork-tender, about 10 minutes depending on the size of your cubes. If needed, add a few tablespoons of water to help cook the sweet potato.

3. Add the shrimp and cook for 2 to 3 minutes, or until it turns pink. Reduce the heat to low and add the kale. Cook, stirring, until wilted. Season with salt and pepper and serve.

*If you don't eat any animal products, you may substitute any vegetarian protein from the Metabolism Revolution Food List on page 56.

Lemon Salmon with Wild Rice

SERVES 1

INGREDIENTS	MEAL MAP A	MEAL MAP B	MEAL MAP C
SALMON*	4 OUNCES	4 OUNCES	8 OUNCES
GROUND PEPPER	AS NEEDED	AS NEEDED	AS NEEDED
DILL, FRESH OR DRIED	½ TEASPOON	½ TEASPOON	1 TEASPOON
LEMON, SLICED	½	½	1
ASPARAGUS	2 CUPS OF 1-INCH PIECES	2 CUPS OF 1-INCH PIECES	2 CUPS OF 1-INCH PIECES
WILD RICE	½ CUP	½ CUP	½ CUP

1. Preheat the broiler on high. Position an oven rack 4 to 5 inches from the heat source. Line a baking sheet with aluminum foil.

2. Place the salmon on the prepared baking sheet. Season the fish with the pepper and dill, and top with the lemon slices. Broil for 10 minutes, or until the fish is opaque and flakes easily with a fork.

3. While the salmon is cooking, steam the asparagus in a steamer or in a steamer basket over boiling water until crisp-tender, about 8 minutes, depending on the thickness of your asparagus.

4. Serve over the wild rice with the asparagus alongside.

*If you don't eat any animal products, you may substitute any vegetarian protein from the Metabolism Revolution Food List on page 56.

Curried Quinoa with Seasoned Pork Medallions

SERVES 1

INGREDIENTS	MEAL MAP A	MEAL MAP B	MEAL MAP C
PORK MEDALLIONS*	4 OUNCES	4 OUNCES	8 OUNCES
SEA SALT AND GROUND PEPPER	AS NEEDED	AS NEEDED	AS NEEDED
QUINOA, RINSED	¼ CUP	¼ CUP	¼ CUP
LEMON ZEST	¼ TEASPOON	¼ TEASPOON	¼ TEASPOON
FRESH LEMON JUICE	1 TEASPOON	1 TEASPOON	1 TEASPOON
CURRY POWDER	⅓ TEASPOON	⅓ TEASPOON	⅓ TEASPOON
BABY SPINACH	2 CUPS	4 CUPS	4 CUPS
SCALLIONS	1 TABLESPOON CHOPPED	1 TABLESPOON CHOPPED	1 TABLESPOON CHOPPED

1. Preheat a grill to medium or heat a grill pan over medium heat.

2. Season the pork with salt and pepper to your preference. Grill for about 5 minutes on each side, or until the internal temperature registers 145°F on an instant-read thermometer.

3. Meanwhile, cook the quinoa according to the package directions, until light and fluffy. Let cool until warm to the touch, then stir in the lemon zest, lemon juice, and curry powder and season with salt and pepper.

4. Put the spinach in a large bowl or on a plate. Top with the quinoa. Place the pork medallions on top of the quinoa and garnish with the scallions.

*If you don't eat any animal products, you may substitute any vegetarian protein from the Metabolism Revolution Food List on page 56.

DINNERS, PART 2

Pistachio Pork
with Broccoli

SERVES 1

INGREDIENTS	MEAL MAP A	MEAL MAP B	MEAL MAP C
OLIVE OIL	2 TEASPOONS	2 TEASPOONS	2 TEASPOONS
BALSAMIC VINEGAR	3/4 TEASPOON	3/4 TEASPOON	1 1/4 TEASPOONS
ONION	2 TABLESPOONS MINCED	2 TABLESPOONS MINCED	1/4 CUP MINCED
GARLIC	1 TEASPOON MINCED	1 TEASPOON MINCED	2 TEASPOONS MINCED
SEA SALT AND GROUND PEPPER	AS NEEDED	AS NEEDED	AS NEEDED
WATER	1 TABLESPOON	1 TABLESPOON	1 TABLESPOON
PISTACHIOS	2 TABLESPOONS CHOPPED	2 TABLESPOONS CHOPPED	2 TABLESPOONS CHOPPED
FRESH CHIVES	1 TEASPOON MINCED	1 TEASPOON MINCED	2 TEASPOONS MINCED
FRESH PARSLEY	1 TEASPOON MINCED	1 TEASPOON MINCED	2 TEASPOONS MINCED
FRESH MINT	1 TEASPOON MINCED	1 TEASPOON MINCED	2 TEASPOONS MINCED
FRESH CILANTRO, CHOPPED	1 TEASPOON	1 TEASPOON	2 TEASPOONS
BROCCOLI FLORETS	2 CUPS	4 CUPS	4 CUPS
PORK CHOP, THICK-CUT*	4 OUNCES	4 OUNCES	8 OUNCES

1. Heat a grill to medium-high or heat a grill pan over medium-high heat.

2. In a medium bowl, whisk together the oil, vinegar, onion, garlic, salt, pepper, and water. Stir in the pistachios, chives, parsley, mint, and cilantro.

3. Steam the broccoli florets in a steamer or in a steamer basket over boiling water until crisp-tender and bright green, about 5 minutes.

4. Lightly oil the grill grate. Grill the pork chop, basting it frequently with half the pistachio marinade; set the other half aside. Grill for 6 to 7 minutes per side, depending on the thickness of the chop, until browned and an instant-read thermometer inserted into the thickest part registers 140°F.

5. Transfer the chop to a plate and drizzle with the reserved pistachio marinade and broccoli. Season with salt and pepper and serve.

*If you don't eat any animal products, you may substitute any vegetarian protein from the Metabolism Revolution Food List on page 56.

Rainbow Chicken and Veggies

SERVES 1

INGREDIENTS	MEAL MAP A	MEAL MAP B	MEAL MAP C
BONELESS, SKINLESS CHICKEN BREAST,* CHOPPED	4 OUNCES	4 OUNCES	8 OUNCES
BELL PEPPER (RED, YELLOW, OR ORANGE)	3/4 CUP CHOPPED	1 1/4 CUPS CHOPPED	1 1/4 CUPS CHOPPED
RED ONION, CHOPPED	1/4	1/4	1/2
ZUCCHINI	1/2 CUP CHOPPED	1 CUP CHOPPED	1 CUP CHOPPED
BROCCOLI FLORETS	3/4 CUP	1 1/4 CUPS	1 1/4 CUPS
OLIVE OIL	2 TABLESPOONS	2 TABLESPOONS	2 TABLESPOONS
SEA SALT	1/4 TEASPOON	1/2 TEASPOON	1/2 TEASPOON
GROUND PEPPER	1/4 TEASPOON	1/2 TEASPOON	1/2 TEASPOON
ITALIAN SEASONING	1/2 TEASPOON	1 TEASPOON	1 TEASPOON
PAPRIKA	1/8 TEASPOON	1/4 TEASPOON	1/4 TEASPOON

1. Preheat the oven to 500°F.

2. Place the chicken, bell pepper, onion, zucchini, and broccoli in a medium roasting dish or rimmed baking sheet. Add the oil, salt, pepper, Italian seasoning, and paprika. Toss to combine. Bake for 15 minutes, or until the veggies are charred and the chicken is cooked through. Serve.

*If you don't eat any animal products, you may substitute any vegetarian protein from the Metabolism Revolution Food List on page 56.

Grilled Steak with Avocado Salsa

SERVES 1

INGREDIENTS	MEAL MAP A	MEAL MAP B	MEAL MAP C
AVOCADO, DICED	¼	¼	¼
RED ONION	2 TABLESPOONS MINCED	2 TABLESPOONS MINCED	2 TABLESPOONS MINCED
JALAPEÑO	1 TEASPOON MINCED	1 TEASPOON MINCED	1 TEASPOON MINCED
FRESH CILANTRO	¾ TEASPOON CHOPPED	¾ TEASPOON CHOPPED	¾ TEASPOON CHOPPED
FRESH LIME JUICE	¾ TEASPOON	¾ TEASPOON	¾ TEASPOON
SEA SALT AND GROUND PEPPER	AS NEEDED	AS NEEDED	AS NEEDED
OLIVE OIL	1 TABLESPOON	1 TABLESPOON	1 TABLESPOON
STEAK*	4 OUNCES	4 OUNCES	8 OUNCES
CAJUN SEASONING	1 TEASPOON	1 TEASPOON	1 TEASPOON
MIXED GREENS	2 CUPS	4 CUPS	4 CUPS
LIME WEDGES	GARNISH	GARNISH	GARNISH

1. In a small bowl, mix the avocado, onion, jalapeño, cilantro, and lime juice and season with salt and pepper to taste. Stir to combine.

2. In a heavy-bottomed skillet, heat the oil over medium-high heat. Add the steak, season with the Cajun seasoning, and cook until slightly blackened, then flip and repeat on the second side, cooking for about 3 to 4 minutes per side for medium-rare, depending on how thick your steak is. When the steak is finished, remove it from the heat and let it rest for 5 minutes.

3. Arrange the greens on a plate. Slice the steak, place it over the greens, and top with the avocado salsa. Garnish with the lime wedges.

*If you don't eat any animal products, you may substitute any vegetarian protein from the Metabolism Revolution Food List on page 56.

Italian Sausage with Roasted Veggies

SERVES 1

INGREDIENTS	MEAL MAP A	MEAL MAP B	MEAL MAP C
CARROT COINS	½ CUP VERY THINLY SLICED	1 CUP VERY THINLY SLICED	1 CUP VERY THINLY SLICED
ZUCCHINI ROUNDS	½ CUP THICKLY SLICED	1 CUP THICKLY SLICED	1 CUP THICKLY SLICED
BROCCOLI	½ CUP CHOPPED	1 CUP CHOPPED	1 CUP CHOPPED
CAULIFLOWER	½ CUP CHOPPED	1 CUP CHOPPED	1 CUP CHOPPED
ONION, THINLY SLICED	¼ CUP	½ CUP	1 CUP
ITALIAN CHICKEN SAUSAGE,* NITRATE-FREE, NO SUGAR ADDED	4 OUNCES	4 OUNCES	8 OUNCES
FRESH BASIL	1 TEASPOON	2 TEASPOONS	2 TEASPOONS
OREGANO, FRESH OR DRIED	1 TEASPOON	2 TEASPOONS	2 TEASPOONS
FRESH PARSLEY, CHOPPED	1 TEASPOON, PLUS A PINCH	2 TEASPOONS, PLUS A PINCH	2 TEASPOONS, PLUS A PINCH
GARLIC POWDER	1 TEASPOON	2 TEASPOONS	2 TEASPOONS
DRIED THYME	¼ TEASPOON	½ TEASPOON	½ TEASPOON
SEA SALT	½ TEASPOON	½ TEASPOON	½ TEASPOON
GROUND PEPPER	¼ TEASPOON	¼ TEASPOON	¼ TEASPOON
OLIVE OIL	2 TABLESPOONS	2 TABLESPOONS	2 TABLESPOONS

1. Preheat oven to 400°F. Line baking sheet with parchment paper.

2. Spread veggies and sausage over the prepared baking sheet. In a small bowl, combine the basil, oregano, parsley, garlic powder, thyme, salt, black pepper, and olive oil. Pour seasoning mixture over veggies and sausage. Toss to coat. Roast for 15 minutes. Toss the veggies and sausage again and roast for 10 to 20 minutes more, or until the veggies are crisp-tender and the sausage is cooked through.

3. Remove from the oven and garnish with the pinch of parsley. Serve.

*If you don't eat any animal products, you may substitute any vegetarian protein from the Metabolism Revolution Food List on page 56.

Chili-Coconut-Lime Chicken with Cauliflower Rice

SERVES 1

INGREDIENTS	MEAL MAP A	MEAL MAP B	MEAL MAP C
COCONUT, UNSWEETENED SHREDDED OR FLAKED OR CHOPPED FRESH	¼ CUP	¼ CUP	¼ CUP
WATER	¼ CUP, PLUS MORE IF NEEDED	¼ CUP, PLUS MORE IF NEEDED	¼ CUP, PLUS MORE IF NEEDED
RED PEPPER FLAKES	PINCH	PINCH	PINCH
LIME, JUICED	¾	1	1
SEA SALT AND GROUND PEPPER	AS NEEDED	AS NEEDED	AS NEEDED
BONELESS, SKINLESS CHICKEN BREAST*	4 OUNCES	4 OUNCES	8 OUNCES
COCONUT OIL	2 TEASPOONS	2 TEASPOONS	2 TEASPOONS
CAULIFLOWER RICE**	2 CUPS	4 CUPS	4 CUPS
FRESH CILANTRO	1 TABLESPOON CHOPPED	2 TABLESPOONS CHOPPED	2 TABLESPOONS CHOPPED

1. In a blender, combine the coconut and water and blend until liquid, adding a little more water if necessary. In a zip-top bag, combine half the coconut mixture, red pepper flakes, half the lime juice, and salt and black pepper to taste, seal the bag, and shake gently to combine. Add the chicken, seal, and shake to coat. Marinate the chicken in the refrigerator for 30 minutes to 1 hour, or up to overnight.

2. When ready to cook, heat a grill to medium-high, heat a grill pan over medium-high heat, or preheat the broiler.

3. Drain the chicken and discard the marinade. Grill or broil the chicken for 4 to 5 minutes on the first side, then 3 to 4 minutes on the second side, depending on its size, until cooked through. Transfer to a plate and let rest for 5 minutes.

4. In a very large skillet, melt the coconut oil over medium-high heat. Add the cauliflower rice, season with salt and black pepper, and cook,

stirring, until tender, 5 to 7 minutes. Stir in the remaining lime juice and add the remaining coconut-water mixture. Add the cilantro and stir to combine.

5. Pile the cauliflower mixture onto a plate and top with the chicken. Serve.

*If you don't eat any animal products, you may substitute any vegetarian protein from the Metabolism Revolution Food List on page 56.

**Many stores sell riced cauliflower in the produce section. If you'd like to make your own, pulse cauliflower florets in a food processor until broken down into rice-size pieces but not mushy.

Lemon Chicken Fettuccine

SERVES 1

INGREDIENTS	MEAL MAP A	MEAL MAP B	MEAL MAP C
SPAGHETTI SQUASH	1	1	1
OLIVE OIL	1 1/2 TABLESPOONS	2 TABLESPOONS	2 TABLESPOONS
BONELESS, SKINLESS CHICKEN BREAST,* CUBED	4 OUNCES	4 OUNCES	8 OUNCES
SEA SALT AND GROUND PEPPER	AS NEEDED	AS NEEDED	AS NEEDED
RED BELL PEPPER	1/2 CUP SLICED	1/2 CUP SLICED	1/2 CUP SLICED
MUSHROOMS	4 OUNCES SLICED	4 OUNCES SLICED	4 OUNCES SLICED
FRESH PARSLEY	2 TABLESPOONS CHOPPED	2 TABLESPOONS CHOPPED	2 TABLESPOONS CHOPPED
LEMON, JUICED	1/4	1/2	1/2
GARLIC	1/2 TEASPOON MINCED	1 TEASPOON MINCED	1 TEASPOON MINCED

1. Preheat the oven to 400°F.

2. Prick the squash all over with a fork and microwave for 5 minutes to soften it. Cut it in half lengthwise, scoop out the seeds, and put the halves in a baking dish, cut-side down. Add 1 tablespoon water and bake for about 40 minutes, or until the squash is tender. Use a fork to scrape the flesh of the squash into long, thin "noodles." You'll need 1 1/2 cups for Meal Map A, or 3 cups for Meal Maps B and C. (You will have more than the amount you need for this recipe, but you could double or triple the recipe, or save the remaining squash to use in another recipe, such as the Spaghetti Squash Stir-Fry on page 188.)

3. In a large skillet, heat 1 tablespoon of the oil over medium heat. Season the chicken with salt and black pepper, add it to the pan, and cook, stirring occasionally, until browned on all sides. Add the bell pepper, mushrooms, and parsley and cook, stirring frequently, for 3 to 4 minutes, until the chicken is cooked through. Add the spaghetti squash noodles and cook, stirring frequently, until heated through. Transfer to a plate.

4. In a medium bowl, combine the remaining ½ tablespoon (or 1 tablespoon for Meal Maps B and C) oil, the lemon juice, and the garlic, season with salt and pepper, and stir until thoroughly mixed.

5. Drizzle the dressing over the pasta mixture and serve.

*If you don't eat any animal products, you may substitute any vegetarian protein from the Metabolism Revolution Food List on page 56.

Almond-Crusted Cod with Ginger Spinach

SERVES 1

INGREDIENTS	MEAL MAP A	MEAL MAP B	MEAL MAP C
OLIVE OIL	1 ½ TABLESPOONS	1 ½ TABLESPOONS	1 ½ TABLESPOONS
BABY SPINACH	2 CUPS	4 CUPS	4 CUPS
FRESH GINGER, PEELED AND GRATED	⅛ INCH PIECE	¼ INCH PIECE	¼ INCH PIECE
SEA SALT AND GROUND PEPPER	AS NEEDED	AS NEEDED	AS NEEDED
COD FILLET*	4 OUNCES	4 OUNCES	8 OUNCES
ALMOND MEAL	2 TABLESPOONS	2 TABLESPOONS	2 TABLESPOONS
FRESH CILANTRO LEAVES	GARNISH	GARNISH	GARNISH
LIME WEDGES	GARNISH	GARNISH	GARNISH

1. In a large nonstick skillet, heat ½ tablespoon of the oil over medium heat. Add the spinach and cook, stirring occasionally, until wilted, 1 to 2 minutes. Set the spinach aside on a plate and wipe out the pan.

2. In the same pan, heat ½ tablespoon of the oil over medium-high heat. Add the ginger and cook, stirring occasionally, for 1 to 2 minutes, or until fragrant. Stir in the spinach and cook for about 1 minute. Season with salt and pepper, transfer to a serving dish, cover to keep warm, and set aside. Wipe out the pan.

3. Pat the cod fillet dry with paper towels and season with salt and pepper on both sides. Place the almond flour on a plate. Coat one side of the fillet in the almond meal.

4. In the same pan, heat the remaining ½ tablespoon oil over medium-high heat. Add the cod, coated-side down, and cook for 3 to 4 minutes or until golden brown. Flip and cook on the second side for 3 to 4 minutes more, until golden brown and cooked through.

5. Transfer the cod to a serving dish and garnish with the cilantro and lime wedges. Serve with the ginger spinach alongside.

*If you don't eat any animal products, you may substitute any vegetarian protein from the Metabolism Revolution Food List on page 56.

Spaghetti Squash Frittata

SERVES 1

INGREDIENTS	MEAL MAP A	MEAL MAP B	MEAL MAP C
SPAGHETTI SQUASH	1	1	1
EGGS*	2	2	2
EGG WHITES*	2	2	2
COCONUT OIL	2 TEASPOONS	2 TEASPOONS	2 TEASPOONS
GARLIC	1/2 TEASPOON MINCED	1/2 TEASPOON MINCED	1/2 TEASPOON MINCED
RED BELL PEPPER	1/4 CUP CHOPPED	1/2 CUP CHOPPED	1/2 CUP CHOPPED
RED ONION	1/2 CUP CHOPPED	1/2 CUP CHOPPED	1/2 CUP CHOPPED
JALAPEÑO	1/2 TEASPOON MINCED	1/2 TEASPOON MINCED	1 TEASPOON MINCED
SPINACH	1/2 CUP	1 1/2 CUPS	1 1/2 CUPS
SEA SALT AND GROUND PEPPER	AS NEEDED	AS NEEDED	AS NEEDED
AVOCADO, SLICED	1/4	1/4	1/4
TURKEY BACON,* NITRATE-FREE	NONE	NONE	4 SLICES

1. Preheat the oven to 400°F.

2. Prick the squash all over with a fork and microwave for 5 minutes to soften it. Cut it in half lengthwise, scoop out the seeds, and put the halves in a baking dish, cut-side down. Add 1 tablespoon water and bake for about 40 minutes, or until the squash is tender. Using a fork, scrape the flesh of the squash into long, thin "noodles." Reduce the oven temperature to 350°F.

3. In a medium bowl, combine the eggs, egg whites, and 1 1/4 cups of the spaghetti squash noodles for Meal Map A or 1 1/2 cups for Meal Maps B and C. Set aside. (You will have more than the amount you need for this recipe, but you could double or triple the recipe, or save the remaining squash to use in another recipe, such as the Spaghetti Squash Stir-Fry on page 188.)

4. In a small oven-safe skillet, melt 1 teaspoon of the coconut oil over medium heat. Add the garlic, bell pepper, onion, jalapeño, and spinach

and cook, stirring occasionally, until the onion and pepper are soft, about 5 minutes. Stir the spinach-pepper mixture into the egg-squash mixture, season with the salt and black pepper, and stir until everything is well incorporated.

5. Coat the same skillet with the remaining 1 teaspoon coconut oil and pour the entire mixture into the skillet. Bake for 20 minutes, or until cooked through in the middle. Remove from the oven and carefully slide the frittata onto a plate using a spatula.

6. Top with the sliced avocado and serve. For Meal Map C, serve with the turkey bacon alongside.

*If you don't eat any animal products, you may substitute any vegetarian protein from the Metabolism Revolution Food List on page 56.

Nutty Chicken

SERVES 1

INGREDIENTS	MEAL MAP A	MEAL MAP B	MEAL MAP C
PECANS	2 TABLESPOONS	2 TABLESPOONS	2 TABLESPOONS
ALMONDS	2 TABLESPOONS	2 TABLESPOONS	2 TABLESPOONS
FRESH BASIL LEAVES	2	2	2
DRIED THYME	¼ TEASPOON	¼ TEASPOON	¼ TEASPOON
DRIED MARJORAM	¼ TEASPOON	¼ TEASPOON	¼ TEASPOON
EGG WHITES*	1	1	1
BONELESS, SKINLESS CHICKEN BREAST* CUT INTO STRIPS	4 OUNCES	4 OUNCES	8 OUNCES
GREEN BEANS	2 CUPS	2 CUPS	2 CUPS
ZUCCHINI	NONE	2 CUPS	2 CUPS
TURKEY BACON,* NITRATE-FREE, COOKED	NONE	NONE	4 SLICES

1. Preheat the oven to 350°F. Line a baking sheet with parchment paper.
2. In a food processor, combine the pecans, almonds, basil, thyme, marjoram, and salt and pepper to taste. Pulse until the mixture is fully combined, moist, and well chopped. Spread the mixture on a plate. Put the egg white in a bowl. Dip the chicken in the egg white to coat, letting any excess drip back into the bowl, then dip it into the nut mixture, completely covering the chicken. Put the coated chicken on the prepared baking sheet. If some of the nut mixture falls off, pat it back on the chicken. Bake for 30 minutes, or until the chicken reaches an internal temperature of 160°F.
3. When the chicken is cooking, steam the green beans (and zucchini if you are following Meal Map B or C) in a steamer or in a steamer basket over boiling water until crisp-tender, about 6 minutes.
4. Serve the chicken with the steamed green beans and, for Meal Maps B and C, zucchini alongside. For Meal Map C, serve the turkey bacon on the side.

*If you don't eat any animal products, you may substitute any vegetarian protein from the Metabolism Revolution Food List on page 56.

Ginger-Citrus Salmon

SERVES 1

INGREDIENTS	MEAL MAP A	MEAL MAP B	MEAL MAP C
OLIVE OIL	1 1/2 TEASPOONS	1 1/2 TEASPOONS	1 1/2 TEASPOONS
BIRCH XYLITOL (OPTIONAL)	1 TEASPOON	1 TEASPOON	1 TEASPOON
FRESH GINGER	1/2 TEASPOON GRATED	1/2 TEASPOON GRATED	1/2 TEASPOON GRATED
FRESH LIME OR LEMON JUICE	2 TABLESPOONS	2 TABLESPOONS	2 TABLESPOONS
SEA SALT	1/2 TEASPOON, PLUS MORE AS NEEDED	1/2 TEASPOON, PLUS MORE AS NEEDED	1/2 TEASPOON, PLUS MORE AS NEEDED
GROUND PEPPER	1/4 TEASPOON	1/4 TEASPOON	1/4 TEASPOON
SALMON FILLET*	4 OUNCES	4 OUNCES	8 OUNCES
BROCCOLI FLORETS	2 CUPS	2 CUPS	2 CUPS
MIXED RED BELL PEPPER AND MUSHROOMS	NONE	2 CUPS SLICED	2 CUPS SLICED

1. In a small bowl, whisk together the oil, birch xylitol, if using, ginger, lime or lemon juice, salt, and black pepper. Pour the marinade into a zip-top bag and add the salmon. Seal the bag and shake to coat the fish. Marinate in the refrigerator for at least 30 minutes or up to overnight, making sure the flesh side of the salmon is soaking in the marinade.

2. When ready to cook, preheat the broiler. Line a baking sheet with parchment paper.

3. Remove the salmon from the bag, reserving the marinade, and place it on the prepared baking sheet skin-side down. Drizzle the marinade over the fish and broil for about 10 minutes, or until the salmon is almost cooked through.

4. While the salmon is cooking, steam the broccoli (and bell pepper–mushroom mixture if you are following Meal Map B or C) in a steamer or steamer basket over boiling water until crisp-tender, about 5 minutes.

5. Transfer to a plate. Serve with the broccoli and, for Meal Maps B and C, the bell pepper and mushrooms.

*If you don't eat any animal products, you may substitute any vegetarian protein from the Metabolism Revolution Food List on page 56.

Spaghetti Squash Stir-Fry

SERVES 1

INGREDIENTS	MEAL MAP A	MEAL MAP B	MEAL MAP C
SPAGHETTI SQUASH	1	1	1
OLIVE OIL	1 TABLESPOON	1 TABLESPOON	1 TABLESPOON
BONELESS, SKINLESS CHICKEN BREAST,* CUT INTO BITE-SIZE PIECES	4 OUNCES	4 OUNCES	8 OUNCES
GREEN BEANS	1/2 CUP HALVED	1/2 CUP HALVED	1/2 CUP HALVED
BELL PEPPER	1/4 CUP DICED	1/2 CUP DICED	1/2 CUP DICED
SCALLIONS	1/4 CUP DICED	1/2 CUP DICED	1/2 CUP DICED
RED PEPPER FLAKES	PINCH	PINCH	PINCH
ZUCCHINI	1/4 CUP SLICED	1/2 CUP SLICED	1/2 CUP SLICED
SEA SALT	1/4 TEASPOON	1/2 TEASPOON	1/2 TEASPOON
PARSLEY, FRESH	1 TEASPOON	2 TEASPOONS	2 TEASPOONS
BASIL, FRESH	1/4 TEASPOON	1/2 TEASPOON	1/2 TEASPOON
SAGE, FRESH OR DRIED	1/4 TEASPOON	1/2 TEASPOON	1/2 TEASPOON
RAW CASHEWS HALVES OR PIECES	2 TABLESPOONS	2 TABLESPOONS	2 TABLESPOONS

1. Preheat the oven to 400°F.

2. Prick the squash all over with a fork and microwave for 5 minutes to soften it. Cut it in half lengthwise, scoop out the seeds, and put the halves in a baking dish, cut-side down. Add 1 tablespoon water and bake for about 40 minutes, or until the squash is tender. Use a fork to scrape the flesh of the squash into long, thin "noodles." Put 1 cup for Meal Map A, or 2 cups for Meal Maps B or C, on a plate and set aside. You will have more than the amount you need for this recipe, but you could double or triple the recipe, or save the remaining squash to use in another recipe, such as the Spaghetti Squash Frittata on page 184.)

3. In a large skillet, heat the oil over medium heat. Add the chicken and green beans, cover, and cook for 3 to 5 minutes. Open the lid and stir. Add the bell pepper, scallions, and red pepper flakes, cover, and cook for 3 to 5 minutes. Open the lid and stir. Add the zucchini, salt, parsley, basil, and sage. Stir to combine everything. Cover and cook until

the chicken is cooked through and the vegetables are tender but not mushy, about 8 minutes.

4. To serve, pour the chicken-vegetable mixture over the spaghetti squash and garnish with the cashews.

*If you don't eat any animal products, you may substitute any vegetarian protein from the Metabolism Revolution Food List on page 56.

Chocolate Mug Cake

SERVES 1

1 egg white
1 ½ tablespoons raw cacao powder
1 ½ tablespoons birch xylitol
4 drops of pure vanilla extract
Dash of sea salt (optional)

1. Put the egg white in a mug and whisk well, then add the cacao, birch xylitol, and vanilla and whisk well to combine.

2. Microwave for 45 to 60 seconds on 50% power. Sprinkle with the sea salt, if desired, and serve.

Note: Mixing all the ingredients in a blender bottle then pouring into a mug works well, too.

You can also bake the mug cake at 350°F for 12 to 15 minutes. Just be sure the mug you use is oven-safe.

Limeade Slushy

SERVES 2

1 lime, peeled
½ teaspoon lime zest
3 packets pure stevia
1 cup water
2 cups crushed ice

Put all the ingredients in a blender, adding the ice last. Blend until smooth and serve.

Easy Lemon Meringues

MAKES 32; SERVES 2

2 large fresh egg whites
1 teaspoon fresh lemon juice
½ cup birch xylitol

1. Preheat the oven to 225°F. Line two baking sheets with parchment paper. Fit a pastry bag with a ½-inch round or star tip (or you can just use a zip-top plastic bag).

2. In a medium bowl using a handheld mixer, beat the egg whites and lemon juice until the whites hold stiff peaks. Beat in the xylitol, 1 tablespoon at a time. Continue beating until the xylitol has fully dissolved (when you rub a bit of the meringue between your fingers, you shouldn't feel any xylitol crystals) and the meringue is very stiff and glossy.

3. Transfer the meringue to the pastry bag (or transfer it to a zip-top plastic bag and snip off a small piece of one corner). Holding the bag perpendicular to the baking sheet, pipe mounds about 2 inches high. Bake for 2 hours, then turn the oven off and leave the meringues in the warm oven overnight. If they're still sticky in the morning, leave them in the oven (or in another dry place) until they are dry. Store any leftovers in an airtight container on the counter for up to two days.

Lemonade Ice Pops

SERVES 6

2 ½ cups cold water
½ cup fresh lemon juice
Pure stevia or birch xylitol (we used 1 ½ tablespoons stevia)

1. Combine the cold water and lemon juice. Sweeten with the stevia or xylitol to taste. Divide the mixture among six ½-cup ice pop molds. Freeze for about 1 hour.

2. Take the pops out of the freezer. Scrape and stir any ice crystals that have formed. Add the ice pop sticks and freeze the pops for 3 to 4 hours more, until solid.

II

KEEP IT
OFF 4
LIFE

7

WOW, THAT WAS FAST.
NOW WHAT?

Youʼve done it. By now, fourteen days have flown by, and you have either polished off those last few pounds, kick-started a major weight loss, or are looking hot for that major event. Your metabolism has been relit and you are burn-baby-burning. Maybe you are ready to maintain that weight loss, but you fear gaining it back if you donʼt do the right thing. Maybe you want to pause and get used to a new lower weight before progressing even further, but you arenʼt sure how to stop losing weight temporarily and get comfortable where you are right now. Or maybe you want to keep at it and lose more than 14 pounds, but youʼre not sure how to keep your awesome momentum going.

What do you do now?

You have many options, depending on whether you are still on your weight loss journey or have reached your goal weight and want to stay there forever. The best diet in the world is no good without follow-up support once you have reached your goal weight. Maybe youʼve seen those weight loss shows where people lose hundreds of pounds, and then you hear on the news a few years later that they have gained all that weight back. That breaks my heart. Anyone who loses a lot of weight needs to know what to do next, or they are at risk of slipping back into old habits and regaining it all again. This does not have to be you. No matter where you are with your weight loss, you can hold steady whenever you want to stop. It's just a matter of understanding how weight maintenance works, and living a lifestyle that is conducive to holding steady at a healthier, more appropriate weight for your body.

The second half of this book is devoted to providing you with a solid and lifelong strategy for maintaining your weight loss, whether you are exactly where you want to be or want to hold steady for a while before losing more. Here are your options.

OPTION ONE: DO IT AGAIN

f you know you have more weight to lose or you have been wildly successful so far and want to keep going, then keep going. The Metabolism Revolution can help you lose up to 14 pounds in fourteen days, but if you have more to lose, you can do it again—up to three times in a row—to lose up to 42 pounds in six weeks. Now that your metabolism is switched into high-gear weight loss mode, you can take advantage of that momentum.

If this is what you decide to do, recalculate your Metabolic Intervention Score at your new current weight. You may still qualify for the same meal map, or you may have shifted to a new one. As your weight keeps ticking downward, redo this calculation so your meal map is always precisely calibrated to your current metabolism. Here is the calculation again:

Metabolic Intervention Score

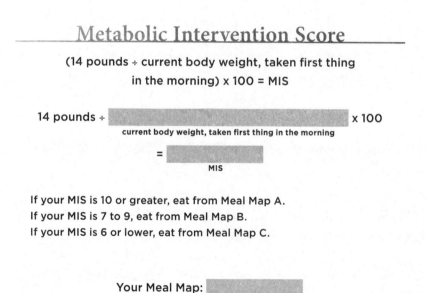

(14 pounds ÷ current body weight, taken first thing
in the morning) x 100 = MIS

14 pounds ÷   x 100
current body weight, taken first thing in the morning

=
MIS

If your MIS is 10 or greater, eat from Meal Map A.
If your MIS is 7 to 9, eat from Meal Map B.
If your MIS is 6 or lower, eat from Meal Map C.

Your Meal Map:

Once you have your new MIS, go back to chapter 4 and start again, following the plan according to your assigned meal map. You might do it exactly the way you did it before, or you might be ready to try some new foods or recipes you didn't try the first time around. Either way, the Metabolism Revolution is here for you.

If you have an even larger amount of weight to lose—say, 75 to 100 pounds or more—then you can take twenty-eight days off before doing another three cycles (use that time to do the 4 Life maintenance program, starting on page 205). As long as you have had a twenty-eight-day break between cycles, you can then go back to the Metabolism Revolution for up to three more cycles. Repeat this as often as you like until you reach your goal weight:

1. Do the Metabolism Revolution for one to three cycles (two to six weeks).
2. Take twenty-eight days off by switching to the 4 Life maintenance program described in detail in the next chapter. (Alternatively, you could do the Fast Metabolism Diet, which is exactly twenty-eight days long.)
3. Go back to the Metabolism Revolution for one to three more cycles (two to six more weeks), for as long as necessary.

OPTION TWO: MIX IT UP

If you still need to lose more weight but you want to mix it up and try something different, I have amazing options for you. Just go to my website at https://hayliepomroy.com/self-discovery-zone and do the self-discovery quiz to see what program will work for you. Switching programs while you are working to lose a larger amount of weight is a good idea to "confuse it to lose it," or cross-train your metabolism. I've got multiple programs specifically tailored to individual desires and issues that you could try—weight loss programs, like the Fast Metabolism Diet; programs to address health issues, such as those in *Fast Metabolism Foods Rx;* and short-term programs to break through weight loss plateaus when your weight stops moving, such as those in *The Burn.* I've also got even more options on my website, like cleanses, intensives, and ongoing challenges, for all kinds of needs. There are not enough pages in one book to cover all the amazing, dynamic aspects of your life, but combine all the interventions I have available to you and you will have the tools to confront every possible weight loss scenario you might encounter, now or in the future, to get your weight to where it needs to be. Once you are there, the 4 Life plan in the next chapter will keep you there.

OPTION THREE: GET COMFORTABLE AT YOUR HOLDING WEIGHT

If you've lost a nice chunk of weight and you feel great, but you still aren't all the way down to your goal, you can hang out at your current weight for a while. Some people feel a little nervous about a new weight they haven't seen in years, or a weight that is below a historical set point they've been trying to get past. If this is you, it can be very valuable to pause right where you are for a while. Even if you still have a lot of weight to go, sometimes it's a good idea to take time to adjust and get comfortable at your new weight—to get it fixed and solid so you feel like it's real. It may not be your ideal weight (yet), but it might be your ideal-for-now weight, and you want to feel strong and solid and confident right there. I call this a holding weight because you are steady and holding, not continuing to lose right now, but not regaining, either.

Let's say you weighed 180 pounds, and now you're down to 166.

Or you haven't been able to get below 200 pounds in years, and now suddenly you are miraculously in the 190s. Those are significant accomplishments, but this weight loss can also be fragile. You can learn to be at a new weight and size and allow your body time to adapt before you go on to lose more. Your psyche may need to catch up to your weight loss. Get used to being a person who is this new, lower weight. Your wardrobe may also need to catch up to your weight loss. Maybe it's time to buy a few new things in a smaller size to celebrate your progress.

Your body may need to catch up to your weight loss. Your skin cells regenerate every two to four weeks. Red blood cells completely replace themselves in four months. The liver renews itself every 150 to 500 days. As your body renews itself at your new, lower, more metabolically active weight, you will feel stronger and more secure. Then, when you are ready, you can begin the process again. Or maybe you will discover that the weight you thought was only temporary feels so good that it actually *is* your ideal weight, after all. There is nothing wrong with adjusting that number in your head.

If you decide to get comfortable where you are, the next chapter will explain the 4 Life maintenance plan, so you can learn to live with a healthy eating plan that will keep your metabolism on fire and keep your weight steady, but will also allow you to live your life without so many restrictions. Stay there until you feel ready and motivated to move on. At that point, you can go back to the Metabolism Revolution to lose another 14 pounds (or more), or try one of my other plans, until you get to where you want to stay for life. Then you can move on to the 4 Life plan permanently.

OPTION FOUR: DONE AND DONE

If you didn't have more than 14 pounds to lose to get to your ideal weight, you might finally be where you have been aiming—your ideal weight. Hooray! I'm so happy for you and so glad to welcome you into our community of successful losers. I designed the 4 Life maintenance plan for you because I know that now that you are here, you don't ever want to go back to that place you were before your Metabolism Revolution.

8

FAST METABOLISM 4 LIFE

hat is maintenance? To understand maintenance from a metabolic perspective, you must understand weight loss from a metabolic perspective. When you are in the process of losing weight, you are changing what the body was doing before when it was gaining weight or holding at a certain weight. You are shaking things loose and getting things moving again. When you feed your body everything it needs and remove elements that were contributing to weight gain and weight loss resistance, your metabolism regenerates and gets hotter and stronger, so that your internal transformation of food into energy becomes more efficient, quicker, and easier. Weight loss is about metabolic movement.

Maintenance, on the other hand, is about holding steady. It is about regaining homeostasis at a new level. You have moved on from where you might have been stuck before (your supposed set point; see page 16), but once you achieve a weight and level of health that you want, your goal is to reestablish stability at this new level. The longer you stay at that weight, the more firmly established your metabolic processes become at that weight. Your body gets accustomed to living there, metabolically, and instead of being weight-loss resistant, you become weight-gain resistant.

Once you are established here, your healed, healthy, strong metabolism can handle some of the things that could have contributed to your weight gain, without shifting beyond about a 5-pound range. A truly healthy metabolism maintains.

Maintenance is the process of getting you firmly established at your new weight so you stay there for life. This won't happen if you bombard your body with metabolic disruptors (see chapter 9), but if you continue to feed it real, good, whole food (with a much broader food list than you were using for weight loss), you keep it moving on a regular basis, and you manage your stress in healthy ways, then when you do encounter the occasional indulgence, your metabolism will burn right through it. You can go to a party and eat a piece of cake, or have a drink, or go to a restaurant, or get sick, or sprain your ankle, or go through a stressful period, and you can bounce right back. That is our goal.

If you've decided you are staying where you are, forever or just for now, the Fast Metabolism 4 Life plan is your new home—a haven from a world full of stress, metabolic disruptors, and temptations that threaten your newly minted fast metabolism.

Is This Phase 4?

If you are already a part of our Fast Metabolism community, you may have heard people talking about "Phase 4." The Fast Metabolism Diet includes three phases each week, with different eating plans in each phase, so you can "confuse it to lose it." That book didn't name Phase 4 as a maintenance phase, but it has become the unofficial designation for how to live after weight loss, which was briefly covered in *The Fast Metabolism Diet* and much expanded upon in conversations online. This chapter systematizes that process for those who have lost weight on the Metabolism Revolution plan or on any of my other plans.

HOW DOES IT WORK?

The Fast Metabolism 4 Life meal plan is a good, sound, strong, healthy nutrition plan for every day, when you aren't working therapeutically on a particular issue. This is a great way to nurture your body and promote longevity and health while preventing disease. You could eat like this for the rest of your life, and eating like this will help you create a healthy life, a happy life, and a life where food is pleasurable. Emotionally, it will also help you establish a healthy relationship with food. It is a style of eating that allows you to get in all your micronutrients. It moves in a rhythm that matches the rhythm of a body with a healthy metabolism, and it is a diet in the best sense of the word—not a "diet" but a D.I.E.T., which in my world means: Did I Eat Today? Eating is and always will be the key to a fast metabolism, and now that you have one, we're going to keep using food to fuel health, success, and a steady weight.

The Fast Metabolism 4 Life plan includes a structure for how to eat most of the time to get all your micronutrients and fuel your life. It also includes a broad and comprehensive food list appropriate for anyone who wants to live a healthy life and maintain their weight. I hope you will explore it by introducing new foods into your diet whenever you can. The more foods you include in your world, the more micronutrients and benefits to you.

But maintenance is about more than food, so I also share my thoughts about:

- How to exercise 4 Life
- How to sleep 4 Life
- How to manage your stress 4 Life
- How to handle the inevitable influence of metabolic disruptors, whether from foods like corn and soy; drinks like coffee and alcohol; obesegens like artificial sweeteners, pesticides, and plas-

tics; and everyday stressors like cold viruses, broken bones, and life stress.

Consider this your foundation. Consider health and a healthy weight to be your new norm. Let's get started living and eating 4 Life.

HEALTHY HABITS 4 LIFE

Living a healthy, balanced life means you aren't on a weight loss plan, but you aren't consistently injuring your metabolism, either. Keep it burning with the healthy habits you have already been practicing on the Metabolism Revolution (or any of my other plans). Here are some habits to practice regularly as part of a healthy life:

1. Keep eating regular, balanced meals—three meals and two or three snacks every day.
2. Eat every 3 to 4 hours. If you wake up at 7:00 A.M. and have breakfast by 7:30, then you can have a snack at 10:30, lunch at 1:30, another snack at 4:30, and dinner at 7:30 P.M. You can adjust this according to your waking time, of course.
3. Always eat breakfast, or at least a snack, within 30 minutes of waking, to light your metabolic fire for the day.
4. Eat and drink only natural whole foods that come from the land, earth, sea, and sky—see the 4 Life Master Food List on page 216 for inspiration and guidance.
5. Reserve grain-based foods for breakfast and dinner, but not lunch. The middle of the day is the peak of your digestive energy, so this is the time to have proteins and fats, which are harder to digest than grains. This also encourages fat burning during the day.
6. Eat fruit at breakfast and lunch, but not after three P.M. This helps stabilize your blood sugar every day.

7. Avoid ingredients you can't pronounce, chemicals, colors, and preservatives. Eat organic, grass-fed, and free-range whenever possible.

8. *Always eat only* nitrate/nitrite-free cured meat products like turkey bacon and sausage, jerky, and deli meat.

9. Exercise five times per week with two rest days, rotating your type of exercise (see page 60).

10. Drink half your body weight in ounces of water every day. Always.

Here is a basic plan for how to organize your food and exercise. You can adapt this structure to your own needs, but this is a great place to start living your healthy, active life while maintaining your weight.

BREAKFAST	A.M. SNACK	LUNCH	P.M. SNACK	DINNER	OPTIONAL EVENING SNACK	EXERCISE
FRUIT	VEGGIE	FAT/ PROTEIN	VEGGIE	FAT/ PROTEIN	VEGGIE	CARDIO (2X/WK)
FAT/ PROTEIN	FAT/ PROTEIN	VEGGIE	FAT/ PROTEIN	VEGGIE	FAT/ PROTEIN	WEIGHT LIFTING (2X/WK)
COMPLEX CARB		FRUIT		OPTIONAL COMPLEX CARB		MIE (1X/ WK)
VEGGIE						REST DAY (2X/WK)

Note: Whenever a meal or snack contains a fat and a protein, there are a few foods that can cover both of these bases in one, such as hummus, nuts and nut butters, whole eggs, and sausage.

Let's take a walk through this meal map and see how it might work for you.

Breakfast: A good balanced breakfast includes a fruit, a fat, a protein, a grain-based carb, and a veggie. You might have a grapefruit, sprouted-grain toast with almond butter (almond butter counts as a fat and a protein), and some cucumber slices; or oatmeal with straw-berries, chicken sausage (fat and protein), and carrot sticks; or scram-bled eggs (fat and protein) and vegetables wrapped in a spelt tortilla with a side of orange slices.

A.M. Snack: A vegetable, a fat, and a protein, like raw veggies with hum-mus or almond butter (both count as a fat and a protein), or chicken slices spread with safflower oil mayo and wrapped in leafy greens.

Lunch: This meal should be grain-free. Focus on a fat, a protein, and a veggie with fruit for dessert. A big salad with salmon and a homemade dressing made with olive oil or a soup with turkey, lots of veggies, and a topping of cubed avocado would be perfect, with mango slices or fresh berries for dessert.

P.M. Snack: Back to a vegetable, a fat, and a protein—maybe naturally cured beef jerky, jicama sticks, and herbed olive oil for dipping.

Dinner: For dinner, choose a fat, a protein, a veggie, and, optionally, a complex carb. Some people find they can add a grain at dinner and not regain any weight. If you have a problem with grains in the eve-ning, you could try a steak, a salad with homemade vinaigrette, and a starchy vegetable like sweet potato, or a vegetable soup with chicken and starchy legumes. Or you could leave off the complex carb if it makes your weight start to creep up.

About Dessert . . .

I am not anti-dessert. But I also know that refined sugar is a me-tabolism killer, and even natural sweeteners put a drag on your metabolism if you overdo them. But when your metabolism is burning hot, you can handle the occasional sweet indulgence. I do have three general rules for desserts, however:

1. *Bake it yourself from real food, or make sure it is made of real food.* I recommend favoring desserts that you make yourself at home using natural sweeteners and whole-grain flours. If you are concerned about your health, you know to avoid refined sugar and flour—there is plenty of research out there demonstrating that these are not only metabolic disruptors, but detrimental to health. Make it at home, and you will know and control everything it contains. As I always say, if you bake it, your metabolism can take it. But if you do eat dessert out there in the world, also confirm it is made with real, actual food.

2. *Be happy when you eat dessert.* It is extremely important to consume desserts only during times of joy and celebration. Desserts spelled backward is STRESSED. If you are loving a dessert ceremoniously or during a time of celebration, your body will metabolize it very differently than it would if you consumed it during a time of stress. Certain hormones and catecholamines are elevated when you are stressed, which can cause the body to hoard that sugar and turn it straight to fat.

3. *Eat fruit first.* If you know you will be eating a dessert, be sure to have fruit for snacks during the day beforehand. Fruit stimulates the enzymes in your body designed to balance the sugar/carb combination typically found in desserts, so your body will be better prepared to metabolize something that accidentally fell into your mouth.

You can find some great desserts here in chapter 11, or for tons more amazing and easy healthy dessert recipes, visit my website, HayliePomroy.com, or my Pinterest page at pinterest.com/hayliepomroy.

4 LIFE EXERCISE

Movement strengthens the body, increases circulation, and encourages healthy organ function, but "exercise" does not mean pounding the pavement every day or boring trips to the gym doing the same routine. As with food, exercise should be varied, so you can get all the benefits from every type. That's why I recommend that you do some cardio, some weight lifting, and some stress-reducing metabolic intervention exercise (see page 62) every week. This a healthy, balanced way to incorporate more movement into your life. You don't have to exercise every day, but you *should* do something physical on most days. Here are my 4 Life Exercise recommendations:

Cardio: 2 or 3 times per week, get your heart rate up to between 120 and 140 beats per minute (bpm) for 20 to 35 minutes. You can do this with any heart-pumping activity you enjoy, like running, cardio machines, cardio classes, swimming, dancing, biking, hiking, sports, stair climbing, or vigorous yoga.

Weights: 2 times per week, lift heavy things. You can weight lift at the gym with a trainer or weight machines to guide you, or at home with dumbbells and maybe a barbell, but get those muscles strong and rotate through all your major muscle groups, like your thigh, butt, calf, chest, abs, back, shoulder, and upper arm muscles. You can also work out these muscles with your own body weight doing calisthenics-style exercises like push-ups, sit-ups, squats, and lunges.

Metabolic Intervention Exercises: At least 1 time per week, do something that moves your circulation without necessarily moving your body. Massage, infrared sauna, acupuncture, Epsom salt baths, dry skin brushing, gentle yoga or stretching, and deep breathing are all great options.

HOW TO MAKE THIS PLAN YOURS

Even when you are "maintaining," there may still be individual issues in your life that make some alterations to the basic 4 Life plan necessary and desirable. Ask yourself: What exactly am I expecting from my food?

If you just want to be nourished, and nourish your family, friends, and loved ones, this nutrient-dense program with amazing recipes will do the trick. But what if you are an athlete? What if you eat out and travel a lot, or tend to party like a rock star? What if exercise isn't an option for you, right now or ever? You can layer in food as a performance enhancer, you can layer in food to compensate for extra stress, and you can layer in food to balance a lack of physical activity. Here's how:

Scenario #1: You Are an Athlete

In my career, I work with a lot of professional athletes, but I also have many clients who work out recreationally to such a degree that I modify their diet, because a recreational athlete is nevertheless an athlete, even if nobody is paying them to do it. To qualify as an athlete requiring a modified food plan, you would have to work out more than five times per week for more than 1 hour at each exercise session. If you are training for a triathlon or a marathon or if the term "gym rat" is one you wear with pride, these modifications probably apply to you. You have to feed yourself like an athlete if you're going to behave like an athlete. Here are your modifications:

1. Within 30 minutes of working out, add an extra fruit portion. The natural sugars in fruit help fuel the metabolic build cycle of muscle and prevent oxygen depletion in the muscle.
2. In the next meal after your workout, increase your protein portion by half. This helps inhibit adrenal stress and supports muscle repair.

For example, let's say you had a veggie omelet and grapefruit for breakfast. In addition to that, on the way to the gym or before your workout, have an apple or a pear. At the next meal post-workout, have six ounces of chicken on a salad instead of four.

Scenario #2: You Party Like a Rock Star (or Just Travel Like One)

Drinking alcohol, staying up late, traveling across the country, and eating out at restaurants frequently are all stressors on the metabolism. If you live like this, I'm not going to tell you to stop. You are who you are. Or maybe your stress is temporary but very real—an intense time at work, a personal or family crisis, or something fun like a trip to Europe or an overly indulgent cruise or resort vacation. All these disruptions create chronic stress and put you at risk for weight regain, but you can help your body manage metabolic disruption like this:

- For two days after a particularly stressful time (like the Monday and Tuesday after a heavy partying weekend, or right after returning from traveling), or for the first two days of every week (or every other week) if your stress is constant and unrelenting, go back to the Metabolism Revolution meal map you did most recently. Follow the Part 1 food plan for two days. The emphasis on fruit and carbs will help soothe and calm your adrenals so they can better handle the stress of your lifestyle. (You can find all these meal maps at the end of this book for easy reference.) I actually have to do this a lot—it's my secret weapon. Just last week I took the red eye on a Friday; worked like crazy out of town all day on Friday, Saturday, and Sunday; and then came home and followed the Part 1 Metabolism Revolution Meal Map A for Monday and Tuesday. This helped me snap right back to my normal routine without feeling drained.
- Alter the snacks on your 4 Life meal plan (see page 293). Instead of the typical snack of vegetable and fat that I recommend (like celery with almond butter), switch to fruit. Fruit is best

for combating stress because it soothes your stress-sensitive adrenals and provides the macronutrients they need to function optimally. Either do this for a few days after a stressful time, or replace at least one snack with fruit per day, every day, if your stress is constant. This is especially crucial when traveling. Take fruit with you—apples and oranges pack well, and big bags of frozen berries or mangoes can defrost slowly in your hotel fridge. It can also be fun to find local fresh fruit at farm stands or markets, depending on where and how you are traveling.

- Totally optional: For really intensive post-stress repair, I have a two-day Weekend Warrior program on my website specifically designed to help you recover from a stressful time, whether negative stress like a work crisis or positive stress like an overindulgent vacation. It includes a Weekend Warrior smoothie, soup, and tea you make at home; all three are specifically designed for recovery.

Scenario #3: Exercise Isn't an Option

Some people can't exercise for physical reasons, either permanent (such as a disability or chronic condition) or temporary (such as after an injury or surgery). Other people won't exercise because they just don't want to exercise. They don't like it and they won't do it. I'm not judging. If you will not be doing exercise, I have a workaround for you.

Follow the 4 Life plan, except on two consecutive days of each week, follow the food plan for Part 2 of the Metabolism Revolution meal map you did most recently. Part 2 on all the meal maps is lower in carbohydrates and contains no grain-based complex carbs. This neatly compensates for a lower level of physical activity. Most people find this is easiest on the first two days of the week, but it can also be a good way to eat on the weekends, especially if that is when you tend to want to overeat carbohydrates. (Find all the meal maps at the end of this book, for easy reference.)

Twice every week, do a Metabolic Intervention Exercise (MIE). As you recall from the first part of this book, these are passive and/or supported activities that increase your circulation without requiring a lot of movement or effort on your part. These are particularly crucial if you are recovering from an injury or surgery. They will speed your healing and ease your stress. But they are also very important for people who never exercise because they accomplish a lot of the same things that exercise accomplishes. They are also quite enjoyable and relaxing. Find the list of MIEs on page 62.

In addition to your MIEs, do two or three minutes twice a day of focused deep breathing. There is a particular type of cortisol burning (burning off the stress hormone) that occurs during cardiovascular exercise that deep breathing seems to mimic, although at a lesser level. Deep breathing lets you use your lungs as your arms and legs. Although this is a good thing for anybody to do, it makes a huge impact for those individuals who cannot or do not exercise. This takes only minutes—you reach a significant benefit at about the seventeenth deep breath.

FAST METABOLISM 4 LIFE MASTER FOOD LIST

I hope this comprehensive list will tempt you to try some new foods and broaden your culinary repertoire. This list is broader and more varied than the Metabolism Revolution food list, because now your metabolism can handle a wider variety of foods that aren't so specifically targeted toward metabolic intervention. You'll get to have many foods you may have missed, and this list should constitute the bulk of the foods you eat every day for the rest of your life.

Of course, not every food you will ever want to eat is on this list. Specifically, I left off metabolic disruptors. I'll talk more about these in the next chapter, but in short, these are the foods that don't support your metabolism. They tend to slow it down, and that's exactly what you want to avoid on maintenance. You want to keep the weight off by keeping your metabolism strong, rather than chipping away at it again. While a strong and hot metabolism can handle the occasional influx of a metabolic disruptor, and those foods don't need to be completely banned forever, they are not on this list because if you do eat them, it should only be occasionally, with discretion.

Of course, these are often the very foods my clients crave after a weight loss plan. The first thing my clients and community usually say to me after they have reached their weight loss goal is "Do I get to have coffee/cookies/ice cream/muffins/tortilla chips/French fries again?" Hey, I want you to live your life. I want you to have fun. Heck, I want to have fun, too. But think very carefully about how you felt before your metabolism revolution—and notice how you feel now. If you gave up coffee, do you remember that searing headache you had for three days? If you gave up sugar, do you remember how sluggish and brain-foggy you felt as your body tried to remove the sugar from your system and calm down the residual inflammation? Do you remember the heartburn, reflux, and/or constipation that no longer bothers you? Do you remember that old number on the scale? Do you remember when you were *not* in a state of homeostasis?

Stick with this list *most of the time* to give your diet structure and to help you keep to the foods that fuel you, rather than slow you down, and you will be okay.

And for those long-term FMDers, note that I have brought back some of the foods that you might be missing . . . like Brazil nuts. Goat cheese. Chocolate. Dates. Green tea. And bananas! (My community will understand when I say I am finally going to take on Bananagate.) These are not on the Master Food List, but they are on an accessory food list I call Foods to Ponder at the end of this chapter. I'm going to tell you exactly how to work them back into your life, if you want them.

Categorizing Conundrum

Oh, the woes of trying to categorize foods. If you have worked with me before on some of my other plans, you will notice that throughout my different food maps, I sometimes change what categories different foods fall into. For example, sometimes sweet potatoes are a vegetable and sometimes they are a complex carb. Sometimes tomatoes are a fruit and sometimes they are a vegetable. This is because my plans focus less on what the food is called and more on the micronutrient values and glycemic impact of the food. Let's stop objectifying food and start paying attention to what food can actually *do for us* at any given moment. I always joke that when my clients ask, "But what does it *count as*?," I say, "Stop profiling your food." I am more concerned about what a food can do for you and how it can help you reach your goal. I refuse to say that a fruit is always a fruit and a vegetable is always a vegetable and a carb is always a carb. What a food is made of and what it can do is what matters, not what we call it. So bear with me on this. The category of a food is less important overall than how you use it to implement the change you need.

FAST METABOLISM 4 LIFE MASTER FOOD LIST

Note that these portion sizes are approximations and ranges. When you are at a healthy weight and your metabolism is humming along, I don't like to tell you exactly how much you should eat, but these represent ranges that work for most people as a portion at any given meal or snack. For information on how you can gauge your own portion needs, see page 245.

VEGETABLES:

minimum 2 cups raw = 1 portion

Artichokes
Asparagus
Bamboo shoots
Beans, all types (green, yellow, wax, and legumes), except soy
Beets, all types
Broccoli, all types
Brussels sprouts
Cabbage, all types
Cactus
Carrots
Cauliflower
Celery, all types
Cucumbers, all types
Cultured/fermented veggies, all types
Eggplant
Fennel
Fiddleheads (coiled fern leaves)
Grape leaves
Hearts of palm
Jerusalem artichoke
Jicama
Kale
Kohlrabi
Leafy greens, all types (lettuces, spinach, kale, etc.)
Leeks
Mushrooms
Okra
Onions, all types
Parsnips
Peppers, all types
Radishes, all types
Rhubarb
Rutabaga
Sea vegetables/seaweeds, all types
Snow peas
Spinach
Spirulina
Sprouts, all types
Squash, all types
Sweet potatoes
Taro
Tomatillos
Tomatoes
Turnips, all types
Wheatgrass
Yucca

FRUITS (FRESH OR FROZEN):

1 to 1 ½ cups or pieces = 1 portion

Apples, all types
Apricots
Berries, all types
Cherimoya
Cherries
Dragon fruit
Figs, fresh only
Grapefruit
Guavas
Jackfruit
Kiwi
Kumquats
Lemons
Limes
Loquats
Lychee
Mangoes
Melons, all type

Nectarines
Oranges, all types
Papayas
Passion fruit
Peaches
Pears, all types
Persimmons
Pineapple
Plantains
Plums

Pluots
Pomegranates
Pomelo
Prickly pears
Quince
Star fruit
Tamarind
Ugli fruit
Watermelon

COMPLEX CARBS:

¼ to ⅔ cup cooked, or 1 slice or piece = 1 portion

Amaranth
Barley, all types
Buckwheat
Einkorn
Farro
Flours made from all approved grains
Freekah
Kamut
Milks made from all approved grains
  (like oat milk)
Millet

Oats (old-fashioned, steel-cut)
Pasta made from all approved grains
Quinoa
Rice, all types except white
Rye
Sorghum
Spelt
Sprouted wheat
Tapioca
Teff
Wheat berries (sprouted)

ANIMAL PROTEIN:

4 to 5 ounces, 2 eggs = 1 portion

Beef
Buffalo
Chicken
Collagen
Cornish game hen
Crustaceans, all types
Cured lean meats, all types (nitrate-free)
Deli meats, all types (nitrate-free)
Eggs
Escargot
Fish, all types (wild-caught, raw,
  smoked, canned)

Frog legs
Gelatin
Jerky, all types (nitrate-free)
Lamb
Mollusks, all types
Organ meats, all types
Pork, all types
Rabbit
Turkey, all types
Wild game, all types

VEGETABLE PROTEIN:

Beans/legumes, all types, except green peas, peanuts, and soy (although vegans who are at their ideal weight and not currently experiencing hormonal issues may choose to eat fermented soy only, on occasion—see more about soy on page 235)

Lentils, all types, ¼–½ cup cooked

Vegetable protein powders (such as from pea, brown rice, etc.—*not soy*), made according to package directions

HEALTHY FATS

Avocado, ¼–½
Cacao butter, 1–2 tbsp
Coconut, fresh or dried (unsweetened), 1–2 tbsp
Hummus, ¼–½ cup
Mayonnaise (made with avocado, olive, safflower, or sunflower oil), 1–2 tbsp

Oils (avocado, coconut, grapeseed, olive, sesame, sunflower, safflower), 1–2 tbsp
Olives, all types, 8–10
Raw nuts and seeds, all types (including raw nut butters, milks, cheeses, and yogurts), 1–2 tbsp

Brazil Nuts and Macadamia Nuts: Green-Lighted

Those of you in my community may recall that I used to say that all raw nuts and seeds were okay, *except Brazil nuts and macadamia nuts.* The reason for this was that it was almost impossible to find either of these nuts in raw form. I didn't want people to miss the importance of eating nuts raw, so I left them off the list. Today, however, probably because the health benefits of raw nuts and seeds have become so much more known, you *can* find raw Brazil and macadamia nuts. Therefore, they are officially back on the list. Just remember: *raw nuts and seeds only.* (Note that all true nuts in their *raw state* are just fine 4 Life, but that does not include peanuts. Peanuts are still a big no—they are actually legumes, not nuts, and I don't ever recommend eating them because they often contain a mold that converts to aflatoxin, a toxic compound linked to liver cancer.)

HERBS, SPICES, CONDIMENTS, AND MISCELLANEOUS FOODS:

Unlimited

Agar

Arrowroot powder

Baking powder

Baking soda

Bragg Liquid Aminos

Brewer's yeast

Broth and stock, all types (homemade or
no sugar added)

Carob (unsweetened)

Chile paste

Coconut aminos

Coconut water

Coffee substitutes (Dandy Blend, Pero)

Cream of tartar

Herbs, all types

Extracts, pure, all types (alcohol-free)

Flavorings and infusions, natural, all
types (alcohol-free)

Guar gum

Herbal teas (caffeine-free)

Hot sauce, all types (no sugar added)

Ketchup (no corn syrup or sugar added)

Liquid smoke

Maca powder

Mustard, all types

Nutritional yeast

Pepper

Pickles (no sugar added)

Raw cacao powder and nibs

Salsa

Sea salt

Spices, all types

Sweeteners, natural (birch-based xylitol,
coconut sugar, pure maple syrup,
molasses, 100% pure monk fruit/lo
han, palm sugar, raw honey, 100%
pure stevia)

Tamari

Vinegars, all types

Water chestnuts

Xanthan gum (non-corn-based)

Zest/peels (citrus)

What's Wrong with Wheat, Corn, and Soy?

I could write a whole book about what agribusiness has done to its three primary staple foods, wheat, corn, and soy (and maybe someday I will). I was an "aggie" in college and studied how agriculture works, including what it does to improve yields and make crops more weather-resistant and profitable. The simple version is that wheat, corn, and soy have all been drastically hybridized over the centuries to increase yield and resistance to weather and pests, and both wheat and corn have also been manipulated to be starchier and sweeter. These hybridization techniques have made these crops more profitable, but at the price of health. Crops resistant to weather and insects are also more resistant to digestion. Crops doused in pesticides and herbicides retain some of those toxic chemicals when you eat them. Crops bred for higher and higher starch and sugar content lose mineral and other nutrient density. Refining those grains into flour or pulling out isolated components (like soy protein isolate or vital wheat gluten or high-fructose corn syrup) increases this effect. Clinically, what I have witnessed is that these three agribusiness products provoke stress-hormone production and tend to cause systemic inflammation in those who eat them. Conventionally grown grain and soy are extremely hard on the body.

As for soy specifically, it is not only heavily sprayed and genetically modified unless it is organic, but even organic varieties contain plant estrogens that may interfere with hormone balance. Soy also contains enzyme inhibitors, a substance called phytic acid that blocks mineral absorption, a clot-promoting substance called hemagglutinin, growth inhibitors, and goitrogens that can interfere with thyroid function.

All that being said, once your metabolism is healed, you can probably handle some of these foods once in a while, but my advice to you is:

• *Instead of wheat*, use organic forms of wheat's distant cousins, spelt, einkorn, and emmer, which have not been manipulated by agribusiness. These and other so-called ancient grains are about to explode in popularity. From behind the scenes, I have been witnessing some major investments into ancient seed banks, and seed clubs and seed preservation societies are popping up everywhere to preserve these ancient grains. Most people don't want to give up grain, but they are becoming more cognizant of the medical health effects of centuries of hybridization and manipulation. This is the answer. There is hope—seeds of change, so to speak, in the right direction. Keep an eye on this trend. Sprouted grain is another option—sprouted wheat is a transformed product because the wheat kernel has sprouted into a plant.

• *Instead of processed corn products*, enjoy organic corn on the cob once in a while. You could also look out for more ancient or heirloom strains of corn and try growing it in your own garden or finding it at your local farmers' market. Corn contains antioxidants and fiber, but pay attention to how it affects you. Corn has a high starch content. If you start eating corn and notice weight gain, this grain may not be for you.

• *Instead of processed soy products,* use only fermented soy, like tempeh, natto, and miso. The fermentation process neutralizes many of the antinutrients and enzyme inhibitors in soy, and if you are a vegetarian or vegan, you will still get the benefits of one of the best protein sources in the plant kingdom. However, as with corn, pay attention to how it affects you. If you gain weight or get hormone-related symptoms, back off the soy. Also, if you are currently experiencing a hormonal shift such as puberty, pregnancy, or menopause, and/or if you have any thyroid dysfunction, avoid all types of soy foods, even organic fermented types.

FOODS TO PONDER

My focus is functional—what can a food do for you? But the truth is that sometimes people just want to enjoy a food purely for pleasure. Can we eat purely for pleasure, not always for function? And if we do, will it compromise the metabolism? I ponder this question. I ponder the idea of food as medicine, as a way to regain and maintain health, as a way to manipulate the body, but I also ponder the notion of food for pleasure.

In particular, I ponder the foods on the following list. These are the foods that keep me up at night, wondering, arguing with myself: Good or bad? Yea or nay? They are not on the 4 Life Master Food List because they aren't particularly good for achieving any specific health or metabolic goal, but I oscillate between using them and not using them only for pleasure. They don't necessarily help your metabolism, but they don't necessarily hurt it, either—in moderation. They all have micronutrient benefits, but they also have the potential for problems in some individuals, and might trigger some people to start overeating again. Ponder, ponder . . . Let's walk through them and discuss. Consider this food for thought.

- ***Bananas:*** I don't hate bananas. In fact, I love bananas. They make an incredible smoothie and a mean ice cream. They are full of potassium and fiber, and make an excellent snack for people who do a lot of cardio. However, I don't include them on any of my food lists, and one of the questions I get asked more than any other is "Why aren't bananas on my food list?" People are very attached to their bananas, as it turns out, and when your metabolism is strong and you are at your goal weight, bananas can be a good dietary choice.

  The problem—the thing that keeps me up at night—is that the banana's high sugar content coupled with its high potassium content tends to make insulin shoot up, which prompts the body to send fat directly to storage without letting cells metabolize it first. If you are prone to insulin resistance or are currently struggling with hormone-based weight loss resistance, or if you are still working on losing weight, bananas can be dicey. Remember my agricultural science background? When farmers need to pack weight onto animals quickly, they give them high-glycemic food (food that raises blood sugar) along with a potassium supplement. They might as well just give them bananas.

  But when your metabolism is on fire and you don't need to lose weight anymore? You should be able to burn right through the occasional banana without an issue. If you do choose to introduce them, consider doing a little banana journal and seeing if adding them to your diet correlates with any weight gain. And try to add them only on those days when you are exercising. That is when bananas can do the most for you.
- ***Chocolate:*** Chocolate is one of those things that worries me. In its raw form, and even in its pure roasted form, it actually has a lot of micronutrients. However, the majority of available chocolate is full of obesegens, from refined sugar to high-glycemic sweet-

eners like high-fructose corn syrup (which they are now allowed to call a "natural sweetener"—but don't you believe it). You can find amazing naturally sweetened raw chocolate products, but they are pricey and rare. The bottom line, I suppose, is to tread lightly and be a savvy label reader. If you are one of those people who lives for chocolate, can you eat it once in a while, or are you better off saying nope, not ever? I believe that pleasure stimulates the metabolism, but obesegens do not, so if you can enjoy an ounce or two of raw naturally sweetened chocolate every week or two and your metabolism is healthy, then this is probably fine.

- *Dried fruit:* Dried fruit contains concentrated micronutrients, and it is a portable snack that, especially in its organic form, packs a ton of energy. When you are getting ready for a high-intensity hike or a cardio session, dried fruit can be a great boost, and it's a good snack for growing children. However, because the drying process concentrates not just the nutrients in the fruit but also the sugars, it drastically increases the fruit's ability to deliver sugar to your body. If you are at your current ideal body weight and your metabolism is humming along, these can be a great addition to your diet. Just proceed with caution and pay attention to how much you are eating, compared to what that fruit would be in its whole form—would you really eat ten pears, fifteen peaches, or a bushel of apples if they weren't dried? Remember that the only difference is the missing water.

- I would also like to call out *dates* specifically, because they are used in so many natural foods as a source of sweetener, such as in smoothies and desserts. Dates are incredibly supportive for thyroid issues, and I love to see them used as part of a healthy diet. Although I would exercise all the same cautions for dates as I do for other dried fruit, I will say that dates are kind of special. Just be careful with them, as they can be snuck into a lot of foods and you can end up eating way more dates than you intend to. If your metabolism starts to struggle, pay attention to how much these are being added to your diet.

- **Grapes:** Non-organic grapes are dirty, dirty, dirty. They are heavily sprayed, and they have also been hybridized to the nth degree. As we know from the wine industry, there are many variations based on soil, but table grapes—the kind most people eat—are particularly high in bioavailable (body-ready) sugars. They should only be eaten in organic form and treated like dessert (see my advice on dessert on page 210).
- **Green peas:** Of all the legumes, these have been hybridized to the hilt, and they vary quite a lot, even from what our grandparents ate. They are one to watch and be suspicious of. A fast metabolism should be able to burn through these quite well on occasion, but if you start adding them and feel like your metabolism is getting a little sluggish—you start gaining weight and feel low on energy—then suspect green peas.
- **Goat and sheep cheese:** Dairy products can be metabolically neutral or metabolic disruptors, depending on their form. Goat and sheep milk are both different from cow milk. Many individuals, particularly kids, who have an allergy to cow milk seem to be able to consume dairy products made with goat or sheep milk. Again, I chalk this up to the influence of agribusiness, which has bred dairy cows for increased milk production, creating commercially raised dairy cows that produce grotesque amounts of milk, which has become more nutrient-poor, with a significant drop in metabolism-enhancing nutrients like CLA, as well as an increase in allergy-stimulating immunoglobulins. Goat and sheep milk both remain much more nutrient-rich and less likely to cause allergic reactions, but I worry that with the popularity of goat and sheep cheese, we might see some of these production practices applied to these animals. And so I fret a little about the future of these products. E-I-E-I-O . . .
- **Potatoes:** Potatoes come in many varieties, and there has been a lot of hybridizing over the centuries. Now there is also genetic modification of potatoes. That means you have a lot of choices. White potatoes tend to have the high glycemic value (they raise

your blood sugar). Most people tolerate purple potatoes the best, and they are beautiful when mashed, combined with hummus, and sprinkled with chives. As with most foods, the more vibrant the color, the more phytonutrients they contain. But white or yellow potatoes? When I'm trying to keep someone's metabolism on fire, you will never hear me suggest to you, my client, that you plop a big old white spud on your plate.

- *Yogurt:* Boy, do you have to be savvy when reading a yogurt label. Sometimes you are better off eating a candy bar. (Not that I'm suggesting you eat a candy bar.) A lot of my clients think they need to eat yogurt for the probiotics, but I would much rather see you getting probiotics from fermented vegetables like kimchi or my fantastic Fermented Salsa (page 293). But if you really love yogurt and you want to eat it, here are my rules of thumb:
  - Goat- and sheep-milk yogurt are better than cow-milk yogurt. My ranking of preference is 1) Goat-milk yogurt, 2) Sheep-milk yogurt, 3) true Greek yogurt with no added sweeteners, binders, or fillers.
  - Yogurt should have a protein-to-carb ratio of at least 1:1, ideally with protein content higher than carb content.
  - Never eat fat-free yogurt.
  - Never eat yogurt with added sugar, food dye, or thickeners.

Ponder those with me, and then note that some of these foods are featured in the recipes in this half of the book, starting on page 261. When they are included, I make a note for you, so you can decide for yourself whether you want to use them. With all the foods on this list, pay close attention. If you are eating some of them and your weight starts creeping up, these are the suspects. Try cutting them out and see if your weight stabilizes again.

Now that you have a plan for yourself, don't forget community. Join us online, where you will get ongoing and continually updated information—there is no nutrition subject I will ever refuse to weigh in on (no pun intended!). Thousands of people out there, worldwide, are doing what you are doing right now, so why not connect? We are all here to help you through the challenges and to celebrate your victories, whether weight-related or NSVs (non-scale victories), like fitting into your skinny jeans again, being able to run around with your grandkids, getting back to a physical activity you love, or finally scoring the brass ring you've always wanted to go for—whether that's your dream job, a life partner, a pregnancy, or just pure joyful self-love.

9

METABOLIC DISRUPTORS: BECAUSE LIFE HAPPENS

They lurk around every corner. They hide in the shadows. They are . . . *metabolic disruptors*. Everything can be humming along fine. Your digestion is efficiently extracting nutrients from the food you eat, and those nutrients are flowing smoothly into your bloodstream and getting nicely absorbed wherever they need to go. Your hormones are balanced. Your liver and lymphatic system are efficiently eliminating waste. You are burning glucose for fuel, and sometimes fat when you need some extra energy, but your fat stores aren't excessive. You have energy. You skin looks good. You sleep well. You enjoy moving. Nothing hurts. You feel contented and happy.

And then. You have a few glasses of wine, or you eat a big slab of cake at a wedding or a birthday party, because . . . cake. You go on vacation and go to town at the buffet . . . every day for a week. Or something negative happens in your life. You lose someone or something. Your job gets really challenging. You fall on the ice and break your foot, or you get the flu.

Your body doesn't just ignore stressors like these. It responds, in an attempt to rescue you. Your digestion may slow down so your body can divert energy to more essential functions. It may also start holding on to fat, in case you need emergency energy later. No matter what you do, you may not be able to burn it. Stress can also cause you to compromise your nutritious diet, and then your body may not be getting all the nutrients it needs to function at peak.

When this happens over a very short period, it's no big deal. A healthy body will quickly recover. But when stress is chronic, your body can't recover so easily. Your metabolism and weight become unstable, and then you might start feeling low on energy, aggressively storing fat and gaining weight, or even feeling unwell.

Metabolic disruptors are a part of life, so what can you do to stay on track 4 Life? Let's identify the main culprits—the metabolic disruptors you are most likely to encounter—so you can be prepared and make decisions with more knowledge.

METABOLIC DISRUPTORS: FOOD AND DRINK

Let's start with the things that I typically don't include in my weight loss plans, but which a healthy metabolism should be able to handle once in a while, in small amounts. In large amounts, or too frequently, these foods and drinks can derail your maintenance because they will slow down your metabolism.

Refined Sugar

Refined sugar is any heavily processed sugar, especially cane sugar (including brown and so-called raw sugar) and high-fructose corn syrup. I also include agave syrup in this category because it is highly refined and concentrated, and brown rice syrup, often used in so-called health foods, because it is also very processed, has no health benefits, and may even contain arsenic.

Sugar may be a quick source of energy, but your body likes to get it from fruit rather than from cane or corn sugar refined beyond recognition. Refined sugar can make it very hard for your body to maintain a stable blood sugar level because it surges into the blood-stream too quickly. When this happens, in order to keep your blood sugar balanced, your body tends to send excess sugar into your fat cells. Just 2 teaspoons of refined sugar can inhibit weight loss for three to four days. One can of soda or one piece of cake or even a modest cookie binge, and you can forget that scale budging for a while, so think about that the next time you are eyeing the dessert cart or lingering in the cookie aisle of the grocery store. On top of all that, roller-coaster blood sugar makes you hungrier, and that can start a chain reaction that can disrupt your stable weight and start it creeping up again. The next time you crave sugar, remember this: The absolute most difficult time to avoid sugar is for the two to three days after eating sugar. If you give in again and again, it will set you up for weight loss resistance. I don't want you to undo all your hard work.

Sugar also suppresses your immune system. Just 2 teaspoons of re-fined sugar can cut your T-cell count by 50 percent for two full hours after eating, leaving you more vulnerable to infection and illness. If you are trying to heal, sugar will make it more difficult.

Finally, know that refined sugar is often combined with a glycopro-tein in processing, meaning it can work its way through the mess of your intestinal tract and into your bloodstream. It's also not a vegetar-ian product, if that is important to you. That glycoprotein comes from bone char or pig's blood, and doesn't have to be disclosed because it is a processing element rather than an ingredient. But, eww.

In short, except for very special situations and under certain con-trolled conditions, treat the white stuff like the profound metabolic disruptor it is. I almost always use pure stevia or birch xylitol when I need an added sweetener.

As for what I do recommend, for weight loss, only use pure stevia or natural birch xylitol, but for maintenance, your metabolism should be able to handle the occasional use of coconut sugar, raw honey, date sugar, or lo han guo.

Refined Wheat Flour ("White Flour")

Refined wheat flour, which can go by many names, including white flour, unbleached wheat four, whole grain wheat flour, etc., is the product of a billion-dollar agricultural business. It has been hybridized far beyond its original form to make it more pest- and weather-resistant, but those genetic changes have also made it more digestion-resistant. Because of this, wheat gives a lot of people a lot of digestive issues, even if they do not have celiac disease (an autoimmune condition that is reactive to gluten, a protein in wheat). People report experiencing many uncomfortable symptoms after eating conventional wheat, such as generalized inflammation as well as gas, bloating, water retention, constipation, stomach pain, diarrhea, fatigue, joint pain, and even neurological symptoms in some people. Wheat is also likely to contain pesticide residue, making it doubly metabolic-disrupting.

The only exception is sprouted wheat bread. When wheat is sprouted into a plant and *then* ground to be used for bread, buns, bagels, or tortillas, it becomes much more digestible to the human body. I include sprouted wheat products in some of my plans, but never conventional wheat or wheat products. That doesn't mean you can't enjoy bread, pasta, or even cookies once in a while. Find sprouted wheat versions, or ones made from any of the far better and more nutrient-dense grains and flours made from them, or from nuts and legumes. Look for bread, pasta, hot cereal, bagels, tortillas, and other snacks made from brown rice, quinoa, amaranth, millet, spelt, and other grains, or from chickpeas, almonds, coconuts, or other non-grain flours. Of course, all these foods are even better if you make them at home.

Coffee (and Caffeine)

Caffeine may feel good in the moment, but it is an extreme adrenal-gland stressor. To have a healthy and fast metabolism, you need your adrenal glands to be strong and functional, because they keep your stress hormone (cortisol) production steady and appropriate, regulate the fight-or-flight hormones (epinephrine and norepinephrine), regulate aldosterone (which controls fat metabolism), help with fat metabolism and sugar storage, and regulate muscle development. When you drink a lot of coffee, you are disrupting all those crucial metabolic functions. You may think coffee is good because it decreases your appetite and helps you to eat less, but remember, *I don't want you to eat less.* I want you to eat *better.*

Also, coffee (including decaf coffee) is one of the dirtiest, most pesticide-laden crops there is. Do you really want to expose your body to all that toxicity first thing in the morning? You are not and never will be caffeine-deficient. Coffee is not an essential food group. But you may be caffeine-addicted. When you give it up, you will have a nasty headache for a few days, and probably some brain fog. Do you want to drink something every day that your body becomes that dependent upon?

There is only one way I will ever even slightly approve of coffee (and even then I have reservations): If you absolutely must have coffee and you are not backing down, please buy the very best organic, low-acid, shade-grown coffee beans. Grind them yourself, brew them yourself, and eat something before you drink the coffee. Coffee on an empty stomach is a metabolism killer.

Soy

You might love it, you might think it is good for you if you are menopausal, and you might rely on it for protein if you are vegan, but in my clinic, *I have never been able to effect true profound weight loss and metabolism repair in someone who is eating a lot of soy food.* Never. I've seen it work for maintenance, but soy is estrogenic in nature, and those plant estrogens love to increase your belly fat. If you *want* belly fat, then soy it up, but otherwise, avoid this stuff like the plague. Why do you think they put soy in livestock feed? Not only does it cheaply increase the protein content, but it also causes rapid weight gain. This is good for the livestock industry, but not for you.

I tell the story in *The Fast Metabolism Diet* of a client I had who was

236 | *METABOLISM REVOLUTION*

an actor. He was very fit, healthy, and trim, but for a role, he needed to look like a chronic alcoholic—bloated, pale, with dark circles under his eyes. I had fourteen days, and I knew what to do. I fed him a bunch of soy, and in just two weeks, he looked like he'd been hitting the bottle hard for years.

While it's true that people in some Asian countries eat soy and many of them are healthy and thin, soy is not actually a major player in the traditional Asian diet. They don't eat it all the time, and they certainly don't eat it in the form of soy protein isolate in a bunch of processed foods. They have small amounts of naturally prepared soybeans or pressed or fermented products (like tofu and miso), mixed with a lot of vegetables and rice. Their soy is also not genetically modified. They also don't have soy mixed into most of their processed food. In fact, the healthiest people in these countries don't eat much, if any, processed food. If you are vegan and you want to eat soy as it occurs in a traditional Asian diet, and you are on maintenance at your ideal weight, and you are not going through a hormonal change right now, you have the green light. Just don't eat it every single day, and stick to strictly organic, non-GMO soy products that are relatively unprocessed, like edamame and tofu, or fermented, like tempeh, miso, and tamari. Fermented organic non-GMO soy has a much lower estrogenic factor and will not slow down your metabolism the same way unfermented soy will.

Alcohol

Let's be straight: Alcohol is a toxin that must be processed by the liver. Is it a fun toxin? It can be, for some people. However, that daily glass (or three) of wine or happy hour margarita will monopolize a major organ of detoxification in your body. (And that margarita is full of refined sugar—see above.) I'm not saying you can never drink alcohol again. But if you do, you may gain a pound or two, and it may take some time for your body to recover metabolically, even from a single drink, and even if you don't have a hangover. If you really want to keep

your metabolism stoked, you will eliminate, or at least limit, your intake of this metabolic disruptor. (See page 247 for some tricks I have
that will help speed along this process, if a margarita or a glass of wine
accidentally falls into your mouth.) If you plan to drink it, do so with
an awareness of what it does to your metabolism.

Dairy

In some forms, dairy products can be nutrient-dense, healthful additions to your diet when added in small amounts, which is why I
included a few of them in the Foods to Ponder list on page 224. But
mainstream, hormone-filled, cheap, refined dairy products like in-
dustrially produced milk and cheese? Nope. Sorry, but the sugar-fat-
protein ratio in cheese and the rate of sugar delivery from the lactose
(milk sugar) in milk are serious metabolism disruptors. Fat-free dairy
products in particular, even when they are organic, aggressively slow
fat metabolism to a grinding halt. Dairy products can also alter your
body's natural production of sex hormones.

Sometimes I use full-fat organic dairy products very strategically
when I am helping women with fertility. Their micronutrients can be
useful for this very specific purpose, but if you are not trying to get
pregnant, or are trying to keep weight off after being pregnant, dairy
should be off your list. Stick with organic unsweetened almond, coconut, rice, or other plant milk instead. They won't disrupt your metabolism the way dairy will.

Corn

Like wheat, corn has been drastically changed through hybridization
over the years, to increase yields and make it taste sweeter. Did you
know that when farmers want to make cows have more marbling (more
fat within the muscle), they feed them a lot of corn before slaughter?
That's what corn does—it is a big chunk of sugar that specifically increases the production of white fat. When I am working with actors

who need to look fat, pregnant, with plump arms, fat cheeks, or round bellies, I feed them corn. When I am working with clients who want to lose weight or maintain lost weight, corn is off the list, including all its sneaky forms, such as:

- Dextrin and maltodextrin, which are derived from cornstarch
- Dextrose, a corn-derived sugar
- Malt, which is not always but often made from cheap corn
- Food starch and modified food starch, also often derived from corn
- Caramel color, often made from corn
- Other ingredients that often contain corn, such as baking powder, vanilla extract made with corn-based alcohol, distilled white vinegar, non-birch xylitol, and iodized salt

4 Life Stress Management

Stress is a part of life. You can't make it disappear. You can't eliminate it from every situation. Typically, most of the energy people expend during times of stress—and that's any type of stress, from emotional to financial to relationship to work stress—is in trying to resolve the stressful situation. But what if you can't? The fact of the matter is that many stressful situations are unresolvable, so instead of trying to end the stress, we need to figure out how to adapt to it and thrive in spite of it.

Stress can be a metabolic disruptor, but I don't include it in the lists in this chapter because it isn't something you can just stop doing. Besides, stress can make you stronger, as long as you get a break from it periodically. The best ways to help your body manage the disrupting influence of chronic stress are to:

- Support the adrenal glands, which regulate stress hormones, by eating nutrient-dense carbs and fruit.

- Keep your blood sugar stable with a steady stream of protein.
- Always eat within 30 minutes of waking.
- Eat every 2 to 4 hours.

It's more important, when you are managing stress, to eat anything—and I do mean anything—than to not eat at all. But obviously, eating something nutrient-rich and supportive is the ideal, so always having adrenal-supporting fruit, micronutrient-rich vegetables, and nitrate-free protein sources on hand will help guide you to the best options.

Supportive techniques can also make a big difference. I am a huge advocate of alternate nostril breathing, essential oil therapy, time spent outside in natural surroundings, and any of the Metabolic Intervention Exercises listed on page 62 for stress management. These can and should become part of your life. They are not luxuries. They are survival techniques.

METABOLIC DISRUPTORS: OBESEGENS/ENDOCRINE DISRUPTORS

Although food is almost always my focus, there are certainly metabolic disruptors in your environment that have nothing to do with what's on your plate. The more you can remove these from your world, the more successful your maintenance (as well as your weight loss) will be:

1. *Toxic cleaning products.* Did you know your choice of cleaning products could be related to the number on your scale? Most conventional cleaning products, from all-purpose cleaning sprays to toilet bowl cleaners, are loaded with fat-soluble toxins, and when your body is bombarded with fat-soluble tox-

ins, it stimulates the creation of more adipocytes (fat cells) to surround those toxins and keep you safe from them. Instead, choose natural cleaning products without artificial ingredients, fragrances, dyes, or preservatives. Fortunately, these are becoming more widely available in stores, and there are hundreds of recipes for natural cleaning products available online, including on my website.

2. *Conventional detergents, soaps, and surfactants.* Look for detergents and soaps made with plant-based ingredients rather than harsh industrial chemicals, and without dyes, fragrances, or preservatives. Especially avoid "antibacterial" soaps, and be aware that "unscented" products often contain secondary chemicals layered on top to remove the smell of the primary chemicals. The only fragrance should be from natural essential oils. Remember, your skin is your largest organ, and when you cover it with chemicals, your body has to metabolize them. And when your body is metabolizing chemicals, it cannot be metabolizing fat.

3. *Masking air fresheners and scented candles.* Your indoor air quality is important. If you are breathing in chemicals, your body has to process them, and when you fill a room with air freshener from sprays, plug-ins, or scented candles, you are filling the air you and your family and pets breathe with chemicals. More work for your liver. Many of these contain potent hormone-disrupting chemicals that have been proven to be dangerous to health, such as phthalates and carcinogens like 1,4-Dichlorobenzene. Air fresheners and scented candles can aggravate asthma and allergies. Rather than cover up smells, use natural cleaning products to eliminate them, and try essential oil diffusers instead of deodorant sprays and plug-ins. Beeswax candles are a good option, too.

4. *Chemical-laced personal care products and cosmetics.* Makeup, shampoo, body lotion, deodorant—anything that goes on your skin can go into your body. Be particularly careful of

anything that goes onto skin where a lot of hair grows—the scalp, underarms, and groin area. These are located near large clusters of lymph nodes—at the base of the skull, under the arms, and in the groin. When you rub these areas with chemicals, you are rubbing them right over your lymph nodes. I bet you never thought what you put under your armpits could affect the scale, but I am telling you that it absolutely does. There are thousands of natural personal-care products, from deodorant and shampoos to cosmetics, available to you, so be a label reader in this area, too. By the way, it is also very important to use natural pads or tampons, or try a reusable silicone cup as a replacement for disposable products during your menstrual period.

5. *Household pesticides and insecticides.* If you need to use herbicides, pesticides, or insecticides at home, on your lawn for weeds, in your kitchen to get rid of ants, or on your pets to control fleas and ticks, be careful. These are potent toxins that can affect indoor air quality and can be acutely dangerous for pets and children, as well as chronically injurious to anyone. There are many natural lawn care companies out there that do not use synthetic chemicals. There are also many nontoxic household insecticide options as well as natural pest-control options for pets (including lots of vacuuming and daily baths with natural pet shampoo containing essential oils rather than synthetic chemicals).

MEDICAL METABOLIC DISRUPTORS

Finally, there are metabolic disruptors you can contract—things like viruses (like Coxsackievirus, Epstein-Barr virus, cytomegalovirus), bacteria (like Lyme disease, chlamydia, staphylococcus, and streptococcus), and fungal infections (like yeast infections, aspergillosis, coccidioidomycosis, histoplasmosis, and ringworm). Some of these can take up residence in your system and actually lower your metabolic rate. If you have one of these infections, or suspect that you do, you will be at greater risk of weight gain or regain. A nutrient-based meal plan along with a healthy, supportive lifestyle is crucial for you, as well as treatment (perhaps from a functional medicine doctor, who is open to therapies beyond the pharmaceutical, when these are effective) to resolve the infection.

Pharmaceuticals you may have to take for chronic conditions can have a negative effect on your metabolism—things like cholesterol medication, antidepressants, prednisone, acid-blocking medication, antianxiety medication, and nonsteroidal anti-inflammatories. If you are prescribed a medication, ask your doctor if weight gain is one of the side effects, and if it is, ask if there are other options that are less likely to have this effect on your metabolic rate.

If you have a diagnosis of a chronic condition, you already know you are struggling. Any inflammatory disorder, autoimmune disorder, blood sugar disorder like diabetes, or other chronic disease diagnosis, as well as any major surgery and/or injury, puts you at a disadvantage. But you already know that, too. Please be compassionate with your body and understand that you need to give yourself permission to support yourself. (I also hope you will check out my book *Fast Metabolism Food Rx* if you are specifically seeking a food plan that can help you deal with a chronic condition. In that book, I talk very specifically about how to nurture a body that is in a diseased state.)

Life happens. You can't avoid stress. You can't avoid some contact with environmental chemicals. You can't avoid change, and sometimes (call me psychic) you are going to eat a food that is a metabolic disruptor just because you really want it.

Fortunately, the 4 Life plan is specifically designed to help your body handle these inevitable life stressors, so sticking to the 4 Life Master Food List most of the time will give your body micronutrient superpowers and will keep your metabolism (and your immune system) highly functional. Keep up with your stress-relieving activities like regular exercise (if you are able), deep breathing, massages, infrared saunas, and meditation, and do your best. Never give up. Health is the journey of a lifetime, and every decision you make for yourself makes a difference.

10

FAST METABOLISM 4 LIFE FAQS

This chapter answers many of the questions my community has asked me about how to live a healthy lifestyle with a fast metabolism. These are 4 Life questions, and I hope yours will be listed here. If you don't see your answer, please come join our smart, supportive community at HayliePomroy.com or come to our Facebook page and ask your questions there.

Q: The portion sizes on the food list are ranges. How do I know exactly how much I should eat?

A: Once you are at a healthy weight and have a healthy metabolism, I don't like to be a dictator about portion size. I give a range because I prefer you to listen to your body. Pay attention to the tangible, measurable signs that give you an indication that your food ratios are in balance:

1. *Monitor your pH.* This can help you determine whether you are getting enough vegetables, in proportion to the amount of protein you are eating. I see this problem a lot in people who have been eating low-carb or in a "paleo" style. They eat a lot of meat and not enough vegetables, and their pH gets too acidic. There is

a lot of data about pH in the membership section of my website. We go over pH testing and walk you through a lemon challenge test. Or you can buy pH strips at any pharmacy for very little cost, and test yourself to see if you are within normal range. If your pH is too acidic, you need to eat more vegetables.

2. *Consider your physical activity level.* When you work your muscles hard (with weight lifting or in the course of your normal day), you usually need more protein. If you do a lot of sustained cardio (running, biking, gym workouts), that can increase your demand for complex carbs and fruit. If you are an athlete, review the modifications I have made for you on page 213.

3. *Make allowances for hormonal imbalance and high cholesterol.* If you are prone to these issues, you should consume higher portions of healthy fats and higher portions of vegetables.

4. *Watch your weight.* The scale is another tangible way to measure whether your portion sizes are off—however, remember that eating less does not mean weighing less. If the scale is creeping up, turn *toward food* for weight loss. Are you having too much of a certain metabolic disruptor? Weight increase is a sign to back off. If you aren't sure of the source of weight creep, you can always circle back to the Metabolism Revolution meal maps for a week or two to get your weight back on track. Do the Metabolic Intervention Score calculation again and follow the meal map linked to your score to get weight gain back under control.

Q: Should I be taking any supplements?

A: Personally, I'm a huge fan of supplements. Targeted micronutrients were an integral part of my being able to get off prednisone and systemic antibiotics as I worked to resolve some serious health issues in my past. I also grew up taking supplements. For me they have been powerful and effective. However, there are a lot of ineffective, mis-represented, dirty products out there in the world of supplements that have been proven to be adulterated with metabolic disruptors. I created my own line of supplements because I wanted something clean and safe and effective for my family, as well as my clients, and I am very choosy about what goes into them. I use them, my kids use them, my clients use them, but you can go with any company you trust to produce a clean product. As for which supplements you should take, everybody's body is specific and everybody's goals are unique. Don't take something if it's not doing what you need, whether supplement or pharmaceutical. Supplements should work hard for you. If you would like to learn more, please explore my website resources on this subject.

Q: I know alcohol is a metabolic disruptor, but I also know I'm going to drink some tonight. Any tips?

A: Sure. As long as you know your liver will take a break from break-ing down fat to process that alcohol, you can do a few things to min-imize the damage:

1. Eat every 3 hours during the day.
2. Eat 10 to 15 grams of protein with every meal and snack.
3. Have a protein snack 30 minutes before you plan to drink. Good options are cocktail shrimp, meatballs, or raw nuts. Avoid empty carbs like chips and cookies.
4. During the event, drink at least 8 ounces of water for every glass of wine, beer, or mixed drink. The water will be even more ef-fective if you add lime juice (not just the wedge—squeeze the wedge, and ask for several).
5. Choose wine or an unsweetened cocktail over beer, which has a much higher carb content.

6. If you are drinking wine, ask for organic, sulfite-free wine. If you are having a cocktail, go for the top-shelf stuff without added chemical ingredients and colors. Clear liquors like gin, rum, vodka, and white tequila are usually purer.

7. Watch mixers. Mixers should not be full of sugar, color, or fake flavor. Soda water is great. Juice should be fresh.

8. The day after, make A Margarita Accidentally Fell into My Mouth Soup (page 302), which is a cleansing and detoxifying broth to help your liver handle the excess load more efficiently. Drink 1 to 3 cups three times during the next day.

Q: Help! The holidays are coming and I don't want to destroy all my hard work, but the foods are so tempting.

A: The holiday season is a challenge when you are trying to maintain weight loss. No question. Many people gain a few pounds during the holidays every year, and that adds up over the years. But that doesn't have to be you. Don't get stressed, though. The holidays should be fun, with a lot of social time with family and friends. Focus on that, and on all the amazing vegetables, fruits, and proteins out there. Be cautious of all the high-fat and high-sugar foods. Try making some of my recipes (in this book, on my website, and on my Pinterest page) that use birch xylitol or 100% pure stevia in place of some or all of the sugar, as well as my many healthy holiday recipes for main dishes and side dishes. Bring your own to social events, and admire but avoid if you can the rich desserts filled with refined sugar and butter. Make your plates colorful and think about how much more fun you will have if you don't feel bloated and guilty. Most of all, have fun. The more you talk, hug, and dance, the less time you will have for hovering over the dessert bar.

I also want to make sure you know that guilt is fattening. Panic is fattening. Stress is fattening. If you can avoid foods that make you feel bad and slow your metabolism, do that. But if you end up indulging in some of them anyway, it's more important not to feel bad about it. Get back on track the next day.

There are also some things you can do to protect yourself and recover afterward, if your face accidentally landed in a plate of Christmas cookies or pumpkin pie.

1. Have breakfast on the day of the holiday or the party. Make sure you have protein.
2. Eat a substantial lunch.
3. Have a fat-based afternoon snack, like nuts, seeds, or avocado. This will help stabilize your blood sugar going in.
4. The day after the party, eat tons of fruits and vegetables to reset, so your indulgence doesn't turn into a season-long binge session. Smoothies are a great way to pack in the produce easily, so start your morning with one of my smoothie recipes (see pages 262 and 295).
5. Afterward, be sure to get back to the basics. Drink half your body weight in water every day. Eat within 30 minutes of waking. Never go more than 4 hours without a meal or snack when you are awake. You know the drill.

Q: I am so stressed out because of something happening in my life. Is there a way to help with food?

A: Of course there is. During times of stress, it is superimportant to focus on healthy carbohydrates, which soothe the body and the adrenals. Eat whole grains instead of refined grains and lots of high-glycemic fruit, like mango, pineapple, watermelon, cantaloupe, and kiwi fruit. Drink lots of natural spring water, sip calming herbal teas like passionflower, ashwagandha, lemon balm, and Siberian ginseng, and eat foods with tryptophan, which helps create calming amino acids. These foods include turkey, legumes, whole grains, nuts, seeds, and cacao (lucky you—chocolate smoothie, anyone? See my recipe on page 295).

Doing more cardio can also really help burn off stress. I also like dry brushing before showering, which gets your lymphatic system moving better. The more efficiently you move toxins out of the body, the less stress you will feel. Deep breathing for a few minutes can calm anxiety, and you may also benefit from listening to some music, stretching for a few minutes, and going to bed early. And I would never stop you from getting a massage. Sometimes a healing touch can make a big difference.

Q: I go out to eat a lot. How do I control what I'm eating in a restaurant?

A: I get this question a lot, and it's a good question because you don't know what's going on in that restaurant kitchen. Many restaurant meals serve huge portions with way more oil, sugar, and salt than you might guess. The best thing to do is plan ahead (see if you can find the menu online), then be very nice to your server when you ask a lot of questions. Explain that you have some dietary restrictions and ask for help. Can items be made without extra sauce, butter, or oil? Can you have veggies as a side instead of potatoes? You can also choose to ignore the bread basket or tortilla chips (or ask the server not to bring it), and focus on vegetables and lean protein when you order.

I always bring tamari packets with me when I eat out. If you ask for something prepared without all the sauce and oil, it can be somewhat tasteless, so this can help you add flavor. You could also ask for lemon or lime wedges. I also often order herbal tea in restaurants, or I bring my own tea bag and flavor my tea with stevia. No, it's not tiramisu, but at least it feels like a special sweet end to the meal. I also always have a bottle of spring water with me. Most restaurants won't care if you bring your own water. (And on special occasions, sure, I'll get the tiramisu, when I'm feeling good and I know my metabolism can handle it.)

Q: I get really hungry when I'm not home. What are easy portable snacks?

A: I call my portable snacks my "crash stash," and they have rescued me on thousands of occasions. Some of my favorites are:

- Fresh fruit, like oranges, tangerines, apples, pears, and kiwis
- Fresh veggies, like a plastic container of cherry tomatoes or a bag of celery sticks or cucumber slices
- Nitrate-free jerky
- Raw almonds, cashews, pecans, pistachios, sunflower seeds, or pumpkin seeds
- Fast Metabolism 4 Life Bars. I always keep a few in my purse.

Q: How do I keep my metabolism fueled when I travel?

A: Traveling can be stressful, and it can also be hard to control your access to good, healthy, pure, whole food. I travel a lot for my job, and I've accumulated some tips. Here's my advice.

- Visit grocery stores instead of convenience stores. You can get fresh fruit, clean protein like nitrate-free deli meat and jerky, and healthy fats like nuts, seeds, hummus, and packets of raw nut and seed butters. Even airports tend to have hummus and veggies these days. Other ideas: tuna pouches; spelt pretzels;

cut-up veggies; and for flavoring plain restaurant food, tamari packets, liquid stevia, balsamic vinegar, small bottles of hot sauce, and small bottles of olive oil.

- Bring an ice chest, if possible. My family invested in one that plugs into our car's cigarette lighter, and we always take it on long car rides. When we plug it in at a hotel, our options are endless.
- My Fast Metabolism shakes and bars are great for traveling when you don't have access to pure food—they're an option.
- Stay hydrated. Drinking a lot of water while traveling is crucial for feeling good, especially during air travel. You can also eat hydrating foods like watermelon, pineapple, and cucumber. Airport kiosks often have these now, too.
- Here are some of the things I always bring with me when I travel:
  - Instant steel-cut oatmeal
  - Stevia sweetener
  - Raw nut butter packets
  - Nitrate-free turkey jerky
  - Fast Metabolism Cleanse Shake
  - A blender bottle
  - Apples
  - Herbal tea packets
  - Cacao nibs
- Every travel day, I drink two cleanse shakes, eat two snacks (typically fruit and nuts, such as an apple with almond butter or mango slices with sunflower seeds), then pick a restaurant that has as clean food as possible and have one meal out per day.
- I also boost my immunity with supplements when I travel—especially with Metabolism Multi, Metabolism Probiotic, Metabolism Enzyme Balance, Metabolism T4T3, and Metabolism Energy, the latter of which is so much better than coffee.

Q: Healthy eating is so expensive. How do I make it more affordable?

A: This is another common question, and it makes me sad that healthy food is so much more expensive than cheap metabolic-disrupting food. But so it goes. Until this changes (and I hope consumer demand will make this happen), try going in on bulk purchases with friends, like meat from local farms and vegetable shares from a CSA or farmers' market. Buy in bulk when good food is on sale, and freeze meat and veggies in meal-specific amounts. Local food is also often cheaper and purer. Check out roadside farm stands, farmers' markets, and u-pick farms. Buy a lot and freeze it. You could also try growing a garden, if you have the space, or a container garden on a patio for things like tomatoes and peppers.

Q: I have a strange work schedule/work at night/work many hours in a row. Does it matter what time I eat? Do I still eat three meals and two snacks or more if I am up for a longer time than most people?

A: Three meals and two snacks is a good place to start, but try to eat every 2 to 4 hours while you are awake, no matter what time of day or night that happens to be. You already know that the first time you eat should be within 30 minutes of waking, even if you sleep during the day and wake up ready for your night shift. This is the time to fuel your metabolism. If you are up for more than 4 hours after finishing your last meal, add an additional snack. That can be first thing in the morning if you like to eat breakfast later, or at the end of the day. The main thing to remember is that whether or not the sun is up, when you are awake, never go more than 4 hours without eating.

Q: I don't have time to cook. Are there frozen or other convenience foods I can use on this plan?

A: Oh, yes. Whether you shop in a health-focused store like Whole Foods, Trader Joe's, or your local food co-op, or you have noticed that your local market has an expanding health food section, you can find a ton of food that will make your food prep easy. Most useful are the many types of frozen vegetables, fruits, and grains, many of which are organic. Look for those with no additives or preservatives. I've also seen more and more frozen precooked meats.

For example, Trader Joe's has a fully-cooked frozen grass-fed beef roast that contains nothing other than grass-fed beef, sea salt, and pepper. The important thing is to become a label reader, because many healthy-looking foods actually aren't. If you see a long list of additives, preservatives, and other chemicals, fillers, and colorings on the label, put it back. If there are no additives, and even better, if the food is organic, grass-fed, pastured, wild-caught, etc., then go ahead and make your life easier.

Better yet, find these foods on sale and buy in bulk. I like to make several pounds of ground beef ahead of time and freeze it in zip-top bags in 1-pound or smaller potions. I will also put a ton of shredded chicken with onions and garlic in the slow cooker and package those portions ahead of time. You could easily cook up enough ground beef and shredded chicken to last you through the entire fourteen-day plan. If you want to eat the same meal for every dinner on Part 1, and the same meal for every dinner on Part 2, then prep gets even easier.

Q: These groceries seem expensive to me, with all the fresh organic produce and meat. Are there ways to make it more affordable?

A: Sometimes I have to get creative with my clients to solve the financial burden of healthy food, but this is a problem that must be solved. We need healthy food to have healthy bodies, and as the market discovers this, it responds. I hope this means that healthy food will only get more available and affordable for all. I see it happening already, as mainstream health consumers are finally discovering that poor-quality food-induced health issues have hit a crisis level, and are demanding better. But until this happens everywhere for everyone, here are some of my favorite strategies for making healthy eating affordable:

- *Buy in bulk, and buy on sale.* If that means getting a large freezer or cooking big batches of things and freezing individual portions once a month, think about how much money you can save with a little more invested effort. Look for the sales and shop around. Find the best deals. Most cities and towns have at least a couple of places to buy food, with rotating sales and more emphasis on "health foods" like organic produce and grass-fed meat, such as one day every month where everything in the health food aisle is on sale. Many stores also have apps that feature deep discount specials for app users only.

  Fortunately, healthy food is becoming more in demand, and that means you don't always have to go to the most expensive stores anymore. In fact, places like Trader Joe's and even Walmart have great deals on organic food. I was at Trader Joe's the other day, and the organic apples were cheaper than the non-organic apples, because they were uglier. Personally, I don't care about ugly. I want apples that will make me healthier, and that's what I want for you, too. And if I can get them for cheap at Walmart, then I will.

- *Find your local farmers' market.* Farmers' markets are an amazing source of fresh local food, often at a cheaper price than the grocery store. To get an even better deal, stop by at the end of the day with cash, when the vendors are in a negotiating mood. I've scored some amazing deals on fresh vegetables and fruits doing this. Many farmers' markets also have locally raised grass-fed beef, pastured pork, and free-range chickens, and even wild-caught fish.

- *Bill your insurance.* Some insurance health savings accounts (HSAs) might cover or reimburse you for the cost of some of your food, if you have a doctor's prescription (written on a prescription pad) for foods related to a particular nutrition plan you are on for your health, especially if you have diabetes or your doctor has told you that you should lose weight. A lot of my clients take my programs to their doctors and can get these prescriptions because the doctors are aware of the results I get with clients whose weight loss is medically necessary. Check with your doctor and your insurance company to see if this might apply to you.

Q: I live in another country, and we have different fruits, vegetables, and fish. How do I do this plan?

A: I find that most people have success with any type of wild-caught fish, and I don't specify fish types on the food list, so enjoy whatever ocean bounty is available to you. As for vegetables and fruits, there is so much variety and diversity across the globe that it would be impossible for me to encompass the options in every country that would be acceptable on this program. Typically, what I recommend for those whose options are different and who can't get the vegetables and fruits listed on this food program is to try to duplicate what is listed. For example, with vegetables, you can substitute leafy greens for leafy greens, or root vegetables for root vegetables for any recipe. With fruits, you could substitute stone fruits for stone fruits, citrus fruits for citrus fruits, or berries for berries. If it seems close in type and color, then you should be fine.

Q: I hate (or my spouse hates) vegetables. I really don't see how I can eat that many. A portion is 2 cups minimum? I don't think so. What can I do?

A: Honestly, the professional advice I have given many of my clients, including those who are internationally famous or have a mind-boggling net worth or who are superstar athletes, is to literally plug their noses if they must. (This is the super-sophisticated method I learned when I had kids.) In all seriousness, though, we must find a way to get those vegetables into you if you want to gain and maintain optimal health, and there are ways to minimize the yuck factor, especially for those of you with super-sensitive taste buds.

- If you don't like a vegetable cooked, try it raw. If you don't like a vegetable raw, try it cooked.
- Get brave and try some vegetables you haven't tried before. Maybe you haven't found your favorites yet.
- Puree vegetables and add them to soup stock, stew, chili, sauce, casserole, or any other savory recipe where you won't notice them or have to experience the texture.
- Throw leafy greens into your smoothies along with some fruit, or raw cacao and fresh mint to mask the flavor.
- Work on desensitizing your palate. Start small, and gradually increase your portions. Break up portions throughout the day. Choose the vegetables you hate the least and then get braver.

Basically, do your best and remember that it is less important to love the taste of every single bite of food you ever take and more important to get the nutrients you need to be healthy. There are unique anti-inflammatory and metabolic-enhancing micronutrients that can only be found in vegetables, gosh darn it. So they need to become part of your life. You can do this.

Q: I have a thyroid issue and I'm not supposed to eat cruciferous vegetables. What are good options for me to get all the vegetables in?

A: There are many vegetable choices on the food lists that are not cruciferous vegetables: asparagus, beets, carrots, cucumbers, green beans, leafy greens, mushrooms, onions, peppers, radishes, and squashes. You can always substitute any vegetable for any other vegetable. Choose those vegetables that aren't cruciferous vegetables (cruciferous vegetables include broccoli, cauliflower, and cabbage). If a recipe you want to try from this book uses cruciferous vegetables, any other vegetable should work, too.

That being said, there is some new thinking about thyroid issues and cruciferous vegetables. When people have thyroid issues, we look at four things: 1) a lack of thyroid hormone production; 2) a lack of conversion from a produced hormone to an active hormone; 3) a dysfunctional conversion from produced hormone to active hormone; and 4) an autoimmunity situation where the body is self-destroying the hormone production site. The cruciferous vegetable debate really only has to do with the dysfunctional conversion problem. What science is now showing us is that typically those individuals have a problem with glutathione metabolism, and that means you don't necessarily need to avoid cruciferous vegetables. What you need to do is make sure you are also eating a lot of antioxidants and selenium-enriched foods. The Metabolism Revolution is heavily weighted toward antioxidants and selenium-rich foods, so you may not need to worry about cruciferous vegetables after all. Talk to your doctor. Or, as I said before, substitute other vegetables for the cruciferous ones, if you're worried. If you want to learn more about this, I have written several blog posts about thyroid issues on my website.

Q: How do I get calcium if I'm not drinking milk?

A: Calcium is a mineral that helps build bone, clot blood, and contract muscles, and also helps the nervous system communicate with the rest of the body. You need about 1,000 mg of calcium every day. People tend to associate calcium with dairy products, but a lot of great foods include calcium, like kale (3 ½ cups have as much calcium as a glass of milk), arugula, broccoli, oranges (1 orange has 60 mg of calcium), sardines (3 ounces with bones has almost 400 mg), salmon, halibut, sesame seeds (3 tablespoons has 280 mg), raw almonds, and legumes like white beans, black beans, chickpeas, kidney beans, and pinto beans. It's easy to get enough calcium when you include these foods in your diet. You don't need dairy products.

Q: I'm pregnant. Do I need to do anything different than follow the standard 4 Life guidelines?

A: Congratulations! What an amazing thing your body is doing right now. The only things I would tell you to do while pregnant are:

1. *Don't diet.* You need a lot of good food to support everything your body is working on.
2. Avoid metabolic disruptors even more stringently than you normally do (they are listed in the previous chapter).
3. Get plenty of protein—specifically, I recommend 60 grams per day during the first trimester, 80 grams per day during the second trimester, and 100 grams per day during the third trimester.
4. Eat lots of healthy fat. Your baby needs omega-3 fatty acids in particular (the kind in fatty fish) for brain development. However, so many larger fish like tuna are contaminated with mercury, it's a good idea to limit your fatty fish consumption to

wild-caught smaller fish only, like sardines, herring, and anchovies. Wild-caught salmon from Alaska and the Pacific coast are also a low mercury risk.

5. Eat tons of fruits and vegetables for their many micronutrients. Enjoy this beautiful time, and with good nutrition, you may even find you have fewer uncomfortable side effects.

Q: I'm nursing a baby. Is there anything particular I should focus on?

A: Yes. Don't worry about weight loss right now. Instead, focus on lots of variety, and especially lots of fruit, which helps keep milk production up and the nutrient quality of your milk high. I generally recommend that nursing moms have five servings of fruit every day.

11

4 LIFE SPECIALTY RECIPES

You can continue to relish any of the Metabolism Revolution recipes you love from chapter 6 while on the 4 Life plan, but you can also expand your horizons with recipes that incorporate new ingredients on the expanded 4 Life Master Food List (see page 218). These recipes take advantage of those foods, including some of the Foods to Ponder I talk about on page 224. Enjoy your new bounty of options.

4 LIFE BREAKFASTS

Blueberry, Avocado, and Coconut Smoothie

SERVES 1

3/4 cup water

1/4 cup coconut kefir

A few ice cubes

1 cup spinach, stems removed

1 cup blueberries

1/4 avocado

Raw cacao nibs

Blend all the ingredients together. Thin with more water if it's too thick, and serve.

Breakfast Banana–Chocolate Chip Bread

SERVES 6

Contains Foods to Ponder: bananas, cocoa powder (optional)

3 overripe small bananas

3 large eggs

¼ cup canned full-fat coconut milk

½ teaspoon pure vanilla extract

2 tablespoons pure maple syrup

½ cup coconut flour

3 tablespoons tapioca flour

2 tablespoons unsweetened cacao or cocoa powder

½ teaspoon baking soda

½ teaspoon baking powder

Pinch of sea salt

¼ cup raw cacao nibs

1. Preheat the oven to 350°F. Line an 9 x 5-inch loaf pan with parchment paper. (You can use a smaller loaf pan if you like a taller loaf, or you could use three muffin tins or ramekins for individual servings.)

2. In a large bowl, mash two of the bananas well and whisk in the eggs, coconut milk, vanilla, and maple syrup.

3. In a smaller bowl, combine the coconut flour, tapioca flour, cacao, if using, baking soda, baking powder, and salt.

4. Fold the dry ingredients into the wet ingredients and stir until everything is fully combined.

5. Cut the third banana into small pieces and fold them into the batter along with the cacao nibs.

6. Pour the mixture into the prepared loaf pan and spread it evenly. Bake for 55 to 60 minutes, until golden brown and a toothpick inserted near the center comes out clean.

7. Remove from the oven and allow to cool completely before cutting into 6 pieces. Wrap any leftovers well and store in the refrigerator for up to 2 days.

Polka-Dot Sweet Potato Bars

SERVES 6

²/₃ cup mashed cooked sweet potato

1 large egg

1 tablespoon coconut oil, melted

1 tablespoon pure maple syrup

2 teaspoons pure vanilla extract

³/₄ cup almond flour or almond meal

³/₄ teaspoon baking powder

³/₄ cup blueberries

1. Preheat the oven to 350°F. Line a 9 x 5-inch loaf pan with parchment paper.

2. In a medium bowl, combine the sweet potato, egg, coconut oil, maple syrup, and vanilla. Whisk with a fork until the mixture looks uniform.

3. In a separate bowl, whisk together the almond flour and baking powder, then stir into the sweet potato mixture until fully combined.

4. Pour the batter into the prepared pan and smooth out the top. Arrange the blueberries on top of the batter, pressing them in just slightly.

5. Bake for 35 to 40 minutes, or until the middle is set. Let cool completely before cutting into 6 pieces. Wrap any leftovers well and store in the refrigerator for up to 2 days.

Nutty Pear Toast

SERVES 1

1 slice sprouted-grain bread
1 tablespoon raw almond butter
½ fresh pear, cored and sliced
1 teaspoon raw honey
1 tablespoon chopped raw almonds or walnuts
Sprinkle of ground cinnamon

Toast the bread as you like it. Spread the almond butter over the toast, top with the pear slices, drizzle with the honey, and sprinkle with the chopped nuts and cinnamon.

Egg and Avocado Breakfast Bowl

SERVES 2

2 scallions, thinly sliced

1 cup cooked quinoa or brown rice

1 teaspoon rice vinegar (unsweetened)

Sea salt and ground pepper

1 tablespoon coconut oil

4 eggs

½ avocado, sliced (optional)

Chili sauce (optional)

½ large or 2 snack-size nori sheets,
cut into thin strips, for garnish

1. In a small bowl, mix together the scallions, quinoa, and vinegar and season with salt and pepper.

2. In a medium nonstick skillet, melt the coconut oil over medium-high heat. Crack the eggs into the skillet, season with salt and pepper, and cook until done to your liking.

3. Divide the quinoa mixture between two bowls. Top each bowl with two eggs and garnish with avocado slices and chili sauce, if desired. Garnish with the nori strips.

Spicy Huevos Rancheros

SERVES 2

3 tablespoons safflower oil

4 scallions, white and light green parts, thinly sliced

1 garlic clove, minced

1 jalapeño or ½ Anaheim pepper, finely chopped (optional;
if you don't like it spicy, add ¼ cup finely chopped green bell pepper)

1 (14.5-ounce) can fire-roasted diced tomatoes

1 cup chopped fresh spinach

¼ cup chopped fresh cilantro

2 (6-inch) sprouted-grain tortillas

2 eggs (any size)

Toppings (use however many of these you want in whatever amount you
want): red and/or green salsa, guacamole, chopped tomatoes

1. Preheat the oven to 375°F.

2. In a medium skillet, heat 2 tablespoons of the safflower oil over medium heat. Add the scallions, garlic, and jalapeño, if using, and cook, stirring continuously, until softened, about 3 minutes. Add the tomatoes, spinach, and cilantro and bring the sauce to a boil. Reduce the heat to medium-low and cover. Cook, stirring occasionally, for about 10 minutes.

3. Meanwhile, put the tortillas in the oven, directly on the rack, and heat just until crisp—this should only take about 10 minutes, more or less, depending on how moist your tortillas are.

4. In a separate nonstick skillet, heat the remaining 1 tablespoon oil over medium heat. Carefully crack the eggs into the skillet and cook them until done to your liking.

5. Remove the tortillas from the oven and put each on a plate. Top each tortilla with half the sauce and an egg. Garnish with any of the desired toppings.

4 LIFE LUNCHES

Tapas Chickpeas with Green Olives

SERVES 4

2 tablespoons safflower oil

1 small red onion, minced

4 garlic cloves, minced

1 (14-ounce) can diced tomatoes

1 tablespoon tomato paste

2/3 cup vegetable broth or fish stock

1 tablespoon red wine vinegar

1 teaspoon smoked or regular paprika

1 teaspoon sea salt

1/2 teaspoon ground pepper

4 sprouted-grain tortillas

1 (14-ounce) can chickpeas, drained and rinsed

1/2 cup green olives, pitted and sliced

1 tablespoon extra-virgin olive oil

Juice of 1 lemon

1/4 cup chopped fresh parsley

1. In a medium skillet, heat the safflower oil over medium heat. Add the onion and cook, stirring, until soft, about 5 minutes, then add the garlic and cook for 2 minutes more. Stir in the diced tomatoes, tomato paste, broth, vinegar, paprika, salt, and pepper. Cover and simmer, stirring occasionally to avoid sticking, for about 15 minutes.

2. Meanwhile, preheat the oven to 400°F.

3. Cut the tortillas into quarters and arrange them on a baking sheet. Toast in the oven until crisp, about 10 minutes (depending on how moist the tortillas are).

4. Uncover the tomato mixture and stir in the chickpeas. Cover and simmer for 5 minutes, or until the chickpeas are heated through. Stir in the olives. Put the mixture in a bowl and drizzle with the olive oil and lemon juice. Sprinkle the parsley over the top and serve with the toasted tortilla wedges (you could also just eat it with a spoon).

Blackened Salmon with Wild Rice

SERVES 4

¼ cup paprika

1 teaspoon cayenne pepper

1 ½ teaspoons thyme, fresh or dried

¾ teaspoon garlic powder

1 teaspoon sea salt

3 ½ tablespoons olive oil

Juice of 1 lemon

4 (6-ounce) salmon fillets

2 cups cooked wild rice

⅓ cup finely chopped fresh parsley

1 lemon, cut into wedges

1. Preheat the oven to 400°F.

2. In a shallow dish (big enough to dip the salmon fillets into), combine the paprika, cayenne, thyme, garlic powder, and ¾ teaspoon of the salt.

3. In a separate shallow dish, combine 2 ½ tablespoons of the oil and the lemon juice. Dip each salmon fillet into the lemon-oil mixture to coat both sides, then coat both sides with the spices.

4. Heat a large oven-safe skillet over medium-high heat. Cook the salmon until blackened, 2 minutes per side.

5. Transfer the pan to the oven and bake for 5 to 8 minutes (depending on the thickness of your fillets), or until the salmon is almost opaque in the center.

6. In a small bowl, combine the wild rice, parsley, remaining 1 tablespoon oil, and remaining ¼ teaspoon salt.

7. Serve the salmon with the rice and lemon wedges alongside.

Garden Turkey Sausage Skillet

SERVES 2

½ pound ground turkey sausage
½ yellow onion, diced
2 garlic cloves, minced
1 cup bite-size pieces zucchini
1 cup bite-size pieces fresh green beans
1 red bell pepper, cut into bite-size pieces
1 (14-ounce) can diced tomatoes
1 teaspoon dried oregano
1 teaspoon sea salt
¼ teaspoon ground pepper
½ cup cherry tomatoes, quartered
½ avocado, cut into cubes

1. Heat a large nonstick skillet over medium-high heat. Add the turkey sausage and onion and cook, breaking up the sausage with a wooden spoon as it cooks, until the sausage is fully cooked and the onion is soft. Add the garlic, stir, and cook for 2 minutes more.

2. Add the zucchini, green beans, bell pepper, tomatoes, oregano, salt, and pepper. Stir until everything is well mixed and cook until the vegetables are tender and brightly colored, about 8 minutes more.

3. Divide the mixture between two plates and top each one with half the cherry tomatoes and half the avocado. Serve immediately.

Warm Butternut Squash White Bean Salad

SERVES 4

¼ cup olive oil

¼ cup white wine vinegar or champagne vinegar

2 garlic cloves, minced

1 teaspoon sea salt

½ teaspoon smoked paprika or chili powder

1 medium butternut squash, peeled, seeded,
and cut into ¾-inch cubes

1 tablespoon safflower oil

1 (14-ounce) can white beans, drained and rinsed

¼ cup raw walnut pieces

8 cups fresh spinach, baby kale, or spring greens

1. Preheat the oven to 425°F.

2. In a small bowl, whisk together the olive oil, vinegar, garlic, salt, and paprika. Set aside.

3. Toss the butternut squash with the safflower oil and spread it over a rimmed baking sheet. Bake until the squash is tender and easily pierced with a fork, about 30 minutes. Transfer the squash to a bowl and immediately add the white beans and the dressing. Toss until everything is fully combined and the beans are warm.

4. Stir in the walnuts and serve over the salad greens.

Tuscan Lunch Soup

SERVES 3

1 tablespoon safflower oil

1 green bell pepper, minced

1 small white onion, minced

2 teaspoons sea salt

1 teaspoon ground pepper

6 garlic cloves, minced

6 slim carrots, sliced

4 cups vegetable broth, plus more as needed

1 (8-ounce) can crushed tomatoes

1 teaspoon dried oregano

½ teaspoon dried thyme

1 (15-ounce) can fava beans or cannellini beans, drained and rinsed

3 cups coarsely chopped kale leaves

2 slices sprouted-grain bread, toasted

1. In a Dutch oven or heavy-bottomed saucepan, heat the safflower oil over medium heat. Add the bell pepper, onion, 1 teaspoon of the salt, and the black pepper. Cook, stirring, until the vegetables are softened, about 8 minutes. Stir in the garlic and cook for 2 minutes more. Stir in the carrots and cook, stirring often, for 8 minutes more.

2. Add the broth, tomatoes, oregano, thyme, and remaining 1 teaspoon salt. Stir everything together and cover. Cook for about 30 minutes, stirring every 5 to 10 minutes to prevent sticking. If the mixture looks dry, add a little more broth or water. After 30 minutes, stir in the beans and kale. Cook, stirring, for 5 minutes more to warm the beans and wilt the kale.

3. Break the toast into bite-size pieces and divide it among four bowls. Ladle the soup over the toast and serve immediately.

Slow Cooker Lentil Power Soup

SERVES 8

2 cups dried green lentils, picked through for stones and rinsed

8 cups vegetable broth

4 celery stalks, finely chopped

4 carrots, thinly sliced

2 leeks, white and light green parts only, thinly sliced and rinsed well

1 yellow onion, chopped

1 (14-ounce) can crushed tomatoes

4 garlic cloves, minced

1 dried bay leaf

2 teaspoons sea salt, plus more as needed

2 teaspoons ground cumin

4 fresh basil leaves, finely chopped

1/2 teaspoon dried thyme

1/2 teaspoon smoked paprika

1/2 teaspoon ground pepper, plus more as needed

4 cups baby spinach

Juice of 1 lemon

1. In a slow cooker or large saucepan, combine all the ingredients except the spinach and lemon juice. Cover and cook on low for about 8 hours (if using a saucepan, cover and cook over low heat for about 4 hours). About 15 minutes before serving, stir in the spinach and lemon juice. Taste and season with additional salt and pepper as needed.

2. Serve warm. This soup will keep in an airtight container in the refrigerator for up to 3 days, or freeze in individual portions for quick meals for later.

Creamy Cauliflower Soup

SERVES 4

6 cups vegetable or chicken broth
1 head cauliflower, cored and chopped into bite-size pieces
1 yellow onion, diced
4 carrots, chopped
2 celery stalks, minced
4 garlic cloves, minced
2 tablespoons minced fresh parsley
2 teaspoons sea salt
1 teaspoon ground thyme
½ teaspoon ground pepper
4 cups coarsely chopped kale leaves

1. In a large saucepan, combine all the ingredients except the kale. Bring to a simmer over medium-high heat, then reduce the heat to medium. Cover and simmer for about 30 minutes, or until all the vegetables are tender.

2. Carefully ladle about half the soup into a blender and blend on low to puree (be careful when blending hot liquids). Return the blended soup to the pot. Stir in the kale and cook for 10 minutes more, or until the kale is wilted.

3. Serve hot. This soup will keep in an airtight container in the refrigerator for up to 3 days, or freeze in individual portions to have an easy meal later.

4 LIFE DINNERS

Smothered Burritos

SERVES 8

½ cup olive oil

5 tablespoons almond flour

⅓ cup chili powder

2 (8-ounce) cans tomato sauce

2 cups water

½ teaspoon ground cumin

½ teaspoon raw cacao powder

½ teaspoon garlic powder

½ teaspoon onion salt

Dash of sea salt

1 (5-pound) pork roast (bone-in) or loin

Sprouted-grain tortillas

Garnishes: fresh cilantro, jalapeño, radishes, avocado, olives, shredded lettuce, almond cheese, and tomato

1. Preheat the oven to 325°F.

2. In a medium saucepan, heat the olive oil over medium heat. Sprinkle the flour and chili powder over the oil and quickly begin to stir. Scrape around the edges of the pan so that all the flour gets incorporated. Simmer for 2 minutes. Slowly add the tomato sauce, water, cumin, cacao powder, garlic powder, onion salt, and sea salt and whisk to combine everything.

3. Simmer over medium heat for 10 minutes. The mixture will reduce and thicken slightly. Remove from the heat and set the enchilada sauce aside.

4. Trim the fat (if any) from the roast. Place the roast in a large slow cooker. Pour all the enchilada sauce over the top. Cover and cook on low for 8 hours, until the pork easily pulls apart with two forks. Scoop out the meat using a slotted spoon. Make sure all the meat is off the

bone (if there is one), grabbing any remaining meat with tongs. Shred the meat.

5. Place 4 ounces of the shredded pork in the middle of a tortilla, add your favorite garnishes, and fold/roll into a burrito. Ladle some sauce from the slow cooker over the top, sprinkle with additional garnishes, and serve.

Baby Bok Stir-Fry

SERVES 2

1 tablespoon grapeseed oil

½ pound ground chicken

1 scallion, chopped, plus more for serving

2 teaspoons grated fresh ginger

2 garlic cloves, finely minced

12 ounces baby bok choy, cut in half

1 tablespoon water

2 teaspoons tamari

2 teaspoons toasted sesame oil

Sesame seeds, for serving

1. In a wok or large sauté pan, heat the grapeseed oil over high heat. Add the ground chicken and cook, stirring, until browned but not fully cooked through. Reduce the heat to medium-high and add the scallion, ginger, and garlic. Cook, stirring, for 30 seconds, or until fragrant.

2. Add the bok choy and water and toss well to coat with the aromatics. Cover the wok. Cook for 2 minutes, or until the bok choy is crisp-tender. Add the tamari and sesame oil and toss well for 30 seconds. The baby bok choy should be just tender in the stem but not too soft. Sprinkle with the sesame seeds and more scallion and serve.

Sweet-and-Sour Salmon

SERVES 2

1 garlic clove, minced
½ teaspoon minced fresh ginger
2 tablespoons tamari
2 tablespoons apple cider vinegar
12 ounces salmon fillet, cut into 2 portions
2 tablespoons raw honey
Pickled ginger slices, for garnish
A few cilantro sprigs, for garnish

1. Preheat the oven to 350°F. Line a rimmed baking sheet with parchment paper.

2. In a bowl, combine the garlic, ginger, tamari, and vinegar. Add the salmon and let marinate for 30 minutes. Put the salmon on the prepared baking sheet, reserving the remaining marinade. Bake for about 15 minutes.

3. Meanwhile, pour the marinade into a small saucepan and bring it to a boil over medium-high heat. Reduce the heat to medium and simmer for about 10 minutes, until the marinade has reduced by half. Remove from the heat.

4. Divide the salmon between two plates. Stir the honey into the marinade and drizzle it over the salmon. Garnish with the pickled ginger and sprigs of cilantro.

Roast Pork with Roots and Fruits

SERVES 4

4 tablespoons safflower oil

1 (16-ounce) pork tenderloin

1 tablespoon dried rosemary

2 1/4 teaspoons sea salt

1 teaspoon ground pepper

1/4 teaspoon ground nutmeg

1 pear, cored and cut into bite-size cubes

1 apple, cored and cut into bite-size cubes

2 sweet potatoes, cut into bite-size cubes

1 yellow onion, cut into bite-size cubes

1 parsnip, peeled and cut into bite-size cubes

6 garlic cloves, root ends sliced off, unpeeled

1 tablespoon olive oil

1. Preheat the oven to 350°F. Grease the bottom of a 9 x 13-inch roasting or baking pan with 2 tablespoons of the safflower oil.

2. Put the pork in the pan and rub it all over with the remaining 2 tablespoons safflower oil.

3. In a small bowl, mix 2 teaspoons of the salt, the pepper, and the nutmeg. Sprinkle half the mixture over the pork and rub it in to coat. Place the pear, apple, sweet potatoes, onion, parsnip, and garlic around the pork and sprinkle with the remaining salt mixture. Bake for 30 minutes.

4. Remove the pork from the oven. Remove the garlic cloves (use tongs to avoid getting burned) and tent the pan with foil. Let rest for about 10 minutes.

5. When the garlic is cool enough to handle, squeeze the roasted garlic into a small bowl. Mix with the olive oil and remaining 1/4 teaspoon salt.

6. Slice the pork into 1/2-inch-thick pieces and place it on a platter (or individual plates). Drizzle with the garlic oil and surround it with the roasted vegetables and fruits. Serve immediately.

Tamari-Ginger Steamed Halibut with Veggies

SERVES 4

¼ cup tamari

¼ cup fresh lime juice

1 tablespoon minced fresh ginger

2 ½ teaspoons minced seeded jalapeño (about 1 small)

½ cup shredded carrot

¼ cup diagonally cut scallions

1 cup sugar snap peas, trimmed

1 cup thinly sliced shiitake mushrooms (about 2 ounces)

1 cup red bell pepper strips (about 1 large)

4 (6-ounce) skinless halibut fillets

8 ounces buckwheat soba noodles

4 tablespoons chopped fresh cilantro

1. Preheat the oven to 425°F.

2. In a wide, shallow dish (big enough to dip the halibut fillets in), whisk together the tamari, lime juice, ginger, and jalapeño and set aside.

3. Tear off four 16 x 12-inch sheets of heavy-duty aluminum foil and fold each in half crosswise. Open the foil and divide the carrot, scallions, snap peas, mushrooms, and bell pepper evenly among the foil sheets.

4. Dip the halibut fillets into the tamari mixture, turning to coat evenly. Place one fillet on each mound of veggies. Spoon the remaining tamari mixture evenly over each serving. Fold the foil over the halibut and veggies and tightly seal the edges. Place the packets on a baking sheet and bake for 13 minutes.

5. Meanwhile, cook the soba noodles according to the package directions, omitting any salt and fat indicated in the directions. Drain and rinse the soba noodles under cold water.

6. Remove the foil packets from the oven and let them stand for 3 minutes.

7. Place 1 cup of the soba noodles on each of four plates and top each with the contents of a foil packet. Sprinkle each serving with 1 tablespoon of cilantro. Serve immediately.

Chipotle Pork Chops

SERVES 4

1 tablespoon chili powder
1 teaspoon paprika
½ teaspoon ground cumin
1 teaspoon ground chipotle
½ teaspoon coarse sea salt
1 garlic clove, minced
4 boneless center-cut pork chops, ¾ to 1 inch thick
2 tablespoons olive oil, or a little more as needed
1 cup canned full-fat coconut milk
1 teaspoon liquid smoke
¼ cup chopped fresh cilantro (optional)
Juice of 1 lime (optional)

1. Heat a large skillet over medium-high heat.

2. In a bowl, combine the chili powder, paprika, cumin, ½ teaspoon of the chipotle, the salt, and the garlic. Brush each pork chop with some of the olive oil, leaving enough for the pan. Rub the pork chops with the spices to coat completely.

3. Coat the skillet with the remaining olive oil and add the pork chops. Cook for 5 minutes per side, or until an instant-read thermometer inserted into the center registers 145°F and the center is only slightly pink. Reduce the heat to low.

4. In a blender or food processor, combine the coconut milk, liquid smoke, cilantro, and remaining ½ teaspoon chipotle and blend until smooth.

5. Pour the sauce over the pork chops. Plate the chops and garnish with the lime juice and extra cilantro, if desired, and serve hot.

Chimichurri Stuffed Salad

SERVES 8

¼ cup olive oil

5 garlic cloves, minced

¼ cup chopped fresh cilantro

¼ cup chopped fresh parsley

½ teaspoon sea salt, plus more as needed

½ teaspoon ground pepper, plus more as needed

Pinch of red pepper flakes

2 pounds flank steak, butterflied

2 hard-boiled eggs, quartered

½ green bell pepper, sliced

½ red bell pepper, sliced

16 cups mixed salad greens

1. Preheat a grill to medium high or preheat the broiler.

2. In a small bowl, mix together the oil, garlic, cilantro, parsley, salt, black pepper, and red pepper flakes. Put the steak on a platter and pour the mixture over the steak, brushing it evenly over the entire surface.

3. Arrange the quartered eggs in three rows across the flank steak at different intervals. Repeat with the sliced bell peppers. Carefully roll up the meat to enclose the filling. Tie the roll with kitchen twine in a few places to hold it together. Season the outside of the roll generously with salt and black pepper.

4. Grill or broil the roll for about 20 minutes, rotating it every 5 minutes. Remove from the grill or broiler and let rest for 15 minutes.

5. Slice the roll, discarding the kitchen twine, and serve over the mixed greens.

Shrimp and Noodle Bowl

SERVES 4

1 tablespoon toasted sesame oil

2 teaspoons grated fresh ginger

2 garlic cloves, minced

¼ cup coconut aminos

1 tablespoon rice vinegar (unsweetened)

6 cups chicken broth

2 cups sliced baby bella (cremini) mushrooms

4 scallions, sliced

1 teaspoon sea salt

4 cups very thinly sliced green cabbage (or use coleslaw mix)

4 cups cooked soba noodles

24 ounces shrimp (any size)

For garnish:

Fresh bean sprouts

Avocado cubes

Chopped fresh cilantro leaves

Very thinly sliced fresh jalapeño

Chopped raw almonds or walnuts

Your favorite hot sauce

1. In a large saucepan, heat the sesame oil over medium-high heat. Add the ginger and garlic and cook, stirring, for 1 minute. Add the coconut aminos, vinegar, and broth. Increase the heat to high and bring to a boil. Reduce the heat to low and simmer, uncovered, for 5 minutes. Add the mushrooms and simmer for 10 minutes more. Stir in the scallions and salt and remove from the heat.

2. Meanwhile, fill a separate pot with water. Bring to a boil over high heat and add the cabbage. Cook for 5 minutes. Stir in the cooked soba noodles and the shrimp. Boil for 2 to 3 minutes more, or until the shrimp are pink. Drain.

3. Divide the noodles, cabbage, and shrimp among four bowls. Ladle the broth into the bowls and garnish with the desired toppings.

Sweet-and-Spicy Meatballs

SERVES 4

2 teaspoons safflower oil

1 pound ground turkey and/or chicken

½ onion, finely chopped

½ cup finely chopped mango

2 garlic cloves, minced

1 tablespoon chopped fresh cilantro

1 tablespoon minced jalapeño
(remove the seeds and ribs for less heat)

2 eggs

½ cup almond flour or coconut flour
(or use Fast Metabolism Baking Mix)

1 teaspoon ground cumin

1 teaspoon sea salt

1 teaspoon ground chipotle or smoked paprika

½ teaspoon ground pepper

1. Preheat the oven to 375°F. Lightly grease a rimmed baking sheet with the safflower oil.

2. Combine all the ingredients in a large bowl and mix well with clean hands. Form into 1-inch balls and arrange in a single layer on the prepared baking sheet. Bake for 20 minutes, or until the meatballs are golden brown and cooked through. Serve hot or enjoy them cold out of the refrigerator as a snack. They will keep in the fridge for up to 2 days, and they also freeze nicely.

4 LIFE DESSERTS

One-Ingredient Banana Ice Cream

SERVES 2

Contains Foods to Ponder: banana

1 very ripe large banana
**Mix-ins of choice, like raw cacao nibs, almond butter,
chopped raw nuts, honey, or ground cinnamon**

1. Peel the banana and slice it. Put it in a zip-top bag, seal, and freeze for at least 2 hours or up to overnight.

2. Put the banana pieces in a small food processor or high-speed blender and blend until the texture resembles soft-serve ice cream. This takes a while, so keep going if you think it's not happening. Add any mix-ins and blend for another few seconds.

3. Transfer to an airtight container and freeze until solid for a more traditional texture, or eat immediately for a softer texture.

No-Bake Gingerbread Cookies

MAKES 18 COOKIES

Contains Foods to Ponder: dates

¼ cup almond meal
¼ cup buckwheat groats
¾ cup gluten-free rolled oats
1 tablespoon ground cinnamon
1 teaspoon ground ginger
½ teaspoon ground nutmeg
¼ teaspoon pure vanilla extract
¼ teaspoon ground cloves
1 ¼ cups packed pitted dates
1 tablespoon coconut sugar (optional)

1. Combine all the ingredients except the dates and coconut sugar in a high-speed blender or food processor and blend until the mixture has a fine consistency, like flour.

2. Add half the dates and blend until well combined, then add the remaining dates and blend until you have a uniform dough.

3. Scoop out rounds of dough about 1 tablespoon in size and roll them into balls, or flatten them with a rolling pin and use a cookie cutter to make desired shapes.

4. Roll the balls in the coconut sugar, if using, or sprinkle the sugar on top of the cookies.

5. For extra chewiness, place the cookies on dehydrator sheets and dehydrate at 115°F for 2 hours. Store in an airtight container on the counter for up to 2 days, or freeze leftovers for later.

Banana Sushi Roll

SERVES 1

Contains Foods to Ponder: bananas

1 firm banana, peeled
2 tablespoons almond or other raw nut butter
1 tablespoon unsweetened shredded coconut
1 tablespoon raw cacao nibs

Spread the banana with the nut butter. Slice it crosswise into bite-size pieces. Roll each piece in the coconut, then in the cacao nibs, pressing them in so they stick. Serve immediately.

Tropical Paradise Chia Pudding

SERVES 2

1 cup canned full-fat coconut milk

½ cup diced fresh or frozen mango

¼ cup chia seeds

**4 drops Metabolism Sweet or other pure liquid stevia,
or 2 teaspoons pure maple syrup**

1 teaspoon lemon zest

1 tablespoon unsweetened coconut flakes

1. In a medium bowl, stir together the coconut milk, mango, chia seeds, stevia, and lemon zest. Cover and refrigerate overnight.

2. In the morning, stir and top with the coconut flakes.

Cacao-Glazed Coin Cookies

MAKES 12 COOKIES

For the cookies

1 1/2 teaspoons coconut oil, melted

1 tablespoon unsweetened almond milk

22 drops Metabolism Sweet or other pure liquid stevia

3/4 teaspoon pure vanilla extract

3/4 cup plus 2 tablespoons almond flour

2 tablespoons raw cacao powder

1/8 teaspoon sea salt

1/8 teaspoon baking soda

For the glaze

1 tablespoon coconut butter, melted

1 teaspoon coconut oil, melted

1/8 teaspoon pure vanilla extract

6 drops pure liquid stevia, or to taste

1 1/2 teaspoons raw cacao powder

1. Make the cookies: In a medium bowl, combine the coconut oil, almond milk, stevia, and vanilla and stir to combine.

2. In a separate bowl, stir together the almond flour, cacao powder, salt, and baking soda.

3. Add the wet ingredients to the dry ingredients and stir well, breaking up clumps as you stir, until you can form the dough into a ball with your hands. Flatten the dough ball into a disk, wrap it in plastic wrap, and refrigerate for 10 minutes.

4. Preheat the oven to 325°F. Line a baking sheet with parchment paper.

5. Place the chilled dough ball between two sheets of parchment paper and roll it out to 1/4 inch thick. Cut 2-inch circles out of the dough

with a cookie or biscuit cutter, transfer to the prepared baking sheet, and freeze for 20 minutes.

6. Bake the cookies for 10 minutes. Remove from the oven and let the cookies cool completely on the baking sheet.

7. Make the glaze: In a small bowl, stir all the glaze ingredients together until smooth.

8. Using a teaspoon, spread a little bit of glaze on each cooled cookie. Store these cookies in an airtight container for up to 2 days, or freeze for later.

Cool and Creamy Mint-Chip Mousse

SERVES 9

1 (14.5-ounce) can full-fat unsweetened coconut milk
½ cup birch xylitol
1 ½ teaspoons pure peppermint extract
1 teaspoon pure vanilla extract
Pinch of sea salt
¼ cup coconut butter, melted
2 ripe avocados
¼ cup raw cacao nibs

1. In a blender, combine the coconut milk, birch xylitol, peppermint extract, vanilla, and salt. Blend to combine.

2. Add the melted coconut butter and the avocados. Blend until creamy.

3. In individual dishes, layer about ¼ cup of the mousse, followed by a scant teaspoon of the cacao nibs, followed by another ¼ cup of the mousse. Garnish with a final sprinkle of cacao nibs.

4. Refrigerate for about 10 minutes before serving. (It's best to serve this right away on the day you make it, since the avocados will gradually lose their green color and turn brown as they oxidize.)

Fermented Salsa

MAKES ABOUT 2 QUARTS

3 pounds tomatoes, chopped
1 red onion, chopped
2 jalapeños, minced
1 cup chopped fresh cilantro
4 garlic cloves, minced
Juice of 2 limes
1 ½ tablespoons sea salt
2 teaspoons ground cumin

1. Combine all the ingredients in a large bowl.

2. Transfer to clean glass jars (leave some room at the top) and cover the jars with a few layers of cheesecloth secured with twine or a rubber band. Leave the salsa on the counter for 2 to 3 days, then screw the lids on tightly and refrigerate. The flavor will continue to intensify in the fridge.

3. Use the salsa as a topping for meats or veggies, or simply eat it on its own. It will keep in the fridge for up to two weeks. It also freezes nicely.

Homemade Beef Jerky

SERVES 4

1 pound organic beef round steak
¼ cup tamari
Juice of 1 lime or lemon
½ teaspoon onion salt
¼ teaspoon garlic powder
¼ teaspoon ground pepper
⅛ teaspoon sea salt
⅛ teaspoon red pepper flakes

1. Trim and discard any fat from the meat. Cut the meat into strips about 5 inches long and ½ inch wide.

2. In a large zip-top plastic bag, combine the tamari, lime juice, onion salt, garlic powder, black pepper, salt, and red pepper flakes. Add the meat to the bag, seal, and toss to coat. Marinate in the refrigerator for at least 8 hours or up to overnight.

3. Drain the meat and discard the marinade. Put the meat on dehydrator sheets (if you have a dehydrator), or line two baking sheets with aluminum foil, set wire racks over the top, and arrange the meat ¼ inch apart on the racks.

4. If you have a dehydrator, dehydrate the meat until it is dry—anywhere from 4 to 12 hours, depending on the temperature and thickness of your meat (follow your dehydrator instructions).

5. If using the oven, preheat the oven to 200°F. Bake the meat, uncovered, for 6 to 7 hours, or until dry and leathery. Remove from the oven and let cool completely.

6. Store the jerky in an airtight container in the refrigerator for up to a week, or freeze it.

4 LIFE THERAPEUTIC/REMEDY/REPAIR RECIPES, FOR WHEN LIFE HAPPENS

Wild Week Repair Smoothie

SERVES 1

Contains Foods to Ponder: dates

Whether you've been stressed out, overworked, or having a ball at a resort or on a cruise, or you're emerging from a decadent holiday weekend of overindulgence, this smoothie will put you right again. Even good times are stressful, and this is just the repair you need. This smoothie is a dream for your adrenals.

¼ cup raw sunflower or pumpkin seeds

1 to 2 cups spinach, kale, or arugula

¾ cup unsweetened coconut milk, rice milk,
or almond milk, plus more as needed

½ cup water

4 or 5 ice cubes

¼ cup frozen cranberries

¼ avocado

1 heaping tablespoon maca

1 tablespoon coconut vinegar or apple cider vinegar

1 unsulfured Medjool date, pitted, or 1 dried fig

2 teaspoons raw cacao powder

2 teaspoons chia seeds

In a blender, pulse the sunflower seeds until they just form a fine powder. Add the remaining ingredients and blend until smooth. Thin with additional water or nondairy milk if desired. Enjoy immediately.

Turmeric Milk

SERVES 2

This golden milk is a delicious, calming before-bed treat that is particularly good if you have pain or inflammation. Turmeric is a powerful anti-inflammatory. Don't skip the pepper—it helps your body absorb the beneficial compounds in the turmeric more efficiently.

2 cups canned full-fat coconut milk or any unsweetened nut milk
1 teaspoon ground turmeric
¼ teaspoon ground pepper
1 (1-inch) piece fresh ginger, peeled and sliced
Raw honey (optional)

1. In a saucepan, whisk together the coconut milk, turmeric, pepper, and ginger. Heat over medium heat until it starts to bubble. Reduce the heat to low and simmer for about 5 minutes.

2. Strain the golden milk into two mugs, add the honey, if desired, and stir. Enjoy immediately.

Chia Elixir

SERVES 1

This elixir is for those queasy tummy or sour stomach days. It corrects pH and absorbs excess acid.

1 tablespoon chia seeds
Juice of ½ lemon
1 tablespoon apple cider vinegar
1 ½ cups warm water

Mix all the ingredients together in a glass. Let stand, stirring occasionally, for 5 to 10 minutes, or until the chia seeds have gelled. Drink up.

Gut-Healing Bone Broth

MAKES ABOUT 12 CUPS

If you have chronic digestive issues, I recommend sipping on this bone broth often and using it as a base for soups you make at home. This is also good for temporary tummy troubles.

4 pounds beef bones

3 bay leaves

1 ½ cups carrots

6 garlic cloves

1 ½ cups sliced leeks

1 onion

3 sprigs rosemary

1 teaspoon whole black peppercorns

2 tablespoons apple cider vinegar

12 cups water

1. Combine all the ingredients in a slow cooker, cover, and cook on low for 6 to 24 hours. Strain the broth, discarding the solids.

2. Drink some immediately and/or freeze the remainder in airtight containers so you always have bone broth on hand to make soup or to make your tummy feel better. It will keep for up to a week in the fridge.

Stress and Anxiety Lemonade

SERVES 12

This lemonade is perfect for relieving anxiety. When you are feeling overwhelmed, have a glass of this. Preferably out on the porch on a beautiful day, but sipping it on the run helps, too.

12 cups water
1 cup raw honey
1 tablespoon culinary-grade dried lavender flowers
Juice of 6 lemons

1. In a large saucepan, combine 6 cups of the water and honey and bring to a boil, stirring to dissolve the honey. Remove from the heat and add the lavender. Cover and let stand for 1 hour. Chill the remaining six cups of water.

2. Strain into a pitcher, discarding the lavender. Stir in the chilled water and the lemon juice. Serve over ice.

PB & J Comfort Food

SERVES 1

This recipe is a surprising remedy for leg cramps . . . and any time you want to feel like a kid again (but without the junk food). And another surprise—you are home-making this jam in about 2 seconds. (But make it the day before.)

2 cups berries, any kind
3 tablespoons raw honey
2 to 3 tablespoons chia seeds
2 tablespoons almond butter
1 slice Ezekiel bread, cut in half

1. In a blender, combine the berries, honey, and chia seeds (use 2 tablespoons for a slightly thinner jam, or 3 tablespoons for a thicker jam). Blend until well combined, transfer to an airtight container, and refrigerate overnight. The chia will gel and set the fruit puree.

2. Spread the chia berry jam on one half of the bread (you won't use it all) and spread the almond butter on the other half. Put the halves together and boom . . . time warp.

Bad Day Mug Cake

SERVES 1

Just one of those crappy days? Cheer yourself up with this chocolaty, minty, crunchy mug cake. Life will seem a whole lot better. This recipe is similar to the Chocolate Mug Cake, but with the refreshing and cheerful addition of mint.

1 egg white
1 ½ tablespoons raw cacao powder
1 ½ tablespoons birch xylitol
1 tablespoon raw cacao nibs
2 drops of pure mint extract
Dash of sea salt (optional)

1. Put the egg white in a mug and whisk well, then whisk in the cacao powder, birch xylitol, cacao nibs, mint extract, and salt, if using.

2. Microwave for 45 to 60 seconds on 50% power.

Note: Mixing all the ingredients into a blender bottle then pouring into a mug works well, too.

You can also bake this at 350°F for 12 to 15 minutes. Just be sure the mug you use is oven-safe.

A Margarita Accidentally Fell into My Mouth Soup

SERVES 8

This recipe will help your liver detox the day after drinking alcohol. It's the best hangover remedy I know.

4 medium zucchini, sliced

1 pound green beans, trimmed and cut in half

2 celery stalks, chopped

Leaves from 2 big bunches parsley, coarsely chopped

Bouquet garni: 1 sprig each of thyme, rosemary, and tarragon, tied together with kitchen twine (optional)

4 cups spring water

Sea salt and black pepper

Combine the vegetables, herb bundle, and water in a large saucepan and bring to a boil. Cover, reduce the heat to low, and simmer for about 30 minutes. Remove the herb bundle. Season with salt and pepper to taste. Eat as is, or puree in a blender.

SUPER-SIMPLE
SUPPORTED PLAN

My community loves to get in the kitchen, share recipes, and find the best ingredients to make metabolism-fueling food, but sometimes that's harder than it sounds. (Or maybe you think it sounds totally hard.) Sometimes, you are busier than usual. Sometimes, you just don't have the energy. Many of my clients and community have expressed interest in a plan that uses my products to minimize cooking even more. If you need an even easier plan than the regular Metabolism Revolution plan, try this Super-Simple Supported Plan, which uses my clean, vegan, whole food–based, micronutrient-rich, anti-inflammatory, and metabolism-supportive Metabolism Meal Replacement Shakes for breakfasts and lunches, along with very easy and portable snacks and the same easy-to-prepare-ahead dinner every night for Part 1, and another every night for Part 2, for both weeks. This streamlines prep and mealtime in a way that will help you get more done in your day when you can't spare a second.

DIANA'S SUPER-SIMPLE SUPPORTED PLAN

Diana is a little bit like Sue (see page 70). She has an extremely busy job as a pharmaceutical rep, so she has very little time to prepare meals. She also travels two or three days or more every week, so she's often nowhere near her kitchen anyway. She really wanted to drop 12 pounds, and her Metabolic Intervention Score put her with Meal Map A, but she told me she couldn't prepare meals every night, and how was she supposed to handle travel? Easy, I told her, and then I showed her this plan—the only information she needed was one model day for her Meal Map A Part 1, and one model day for her Meal Map A Part 2. Every day of Part 1 (the first four days of each week, according to the Meal Map A 4/3 split), she would eat the same thing—a Metabolism Meal Replacement Shake for breakfast, a simple portable snack in the midmorning, another shake for lunch, a simple afternoon snack, and a Part 1 dinner.

She would do the same thing in Part 2, but with compliant snacks and a Part 2 dinner. I explained that she could spend one day—just one—preparing the two recipes. All she had to do was make eight portions of her chosen Part 1 dinner and six portions of her chosen Part 2 dinner. She admitted she had a free Sunday, and she spent only two hours making the recipes. She packed up the week 1 meals into individual portions in the refrigerator, and packed up the week 2 meals in individual portions for the freezer. She found a shaker bottle and I showed her how to portion out her shakes in zip-top bags for travel. All she needed was a bottle of spring water for each shake, something she could easily purchase on the road.

Diana reported back to me that it was easier than she thought it would be. She was able to keep her preprepared dinners in a cooler and even heat them in a hotel microwave when she was driving; once she even packed two frozen dinners in her suitcase for a flight. Her snacks were easy to keep in her purse, and the shakes went with her everywhere. She loved being able to pour, shake, drink, and be done with her meal. And by the end of the fourteen days? *Thirteen pounds down.* Now Diana lives the Fast Metabolism 4 Life lifestyle (see page 205) and a year later, she's still at her ideal weight and holding.

Here is exactly what she did. Note that this meal map contains the two dinners Diana chose, but you could choose any Part 1 recipe and any Part 2 recipe to make ahead for your dinners. You could also make more than one dinner, if you have the time. Just be sure it coincides with the correct part and that you prepare it in the amount appropriate for Meal Map A.

(Note that weight, water, and exercise are not included in this sample meal map, but Diana tracked them, and you should, too, on your blank meal map following page 313.)

SUPER-SIMPLE SUPPORTED PLAN FOR MEAL MAP A: DIANA (Recipes start on page 123.)

	BREAKFAST	A.M. SNACK	LUNCH	P.M. SNACK	DINNER
PART 1 (MONDAY–THURSDAY)	METABOLISM MEAL REPLACEMENT SHAKE: 1½ SCOOPS	ORANGE	METABOLISM MEAL REPLACEMENT SHAKE: 1½ SCOOPS	1 CUP BERRIES	STEAK AND QUINOA BOWL
PART 2 (FRIDAY–SUNDAY)	METABOLISM MEAL REPLACEMENT SHAKE: 1½ SCOOPS	APPLE WITH 2 TABLESPOONS ALMOND BUTTER (IN TRAVEL-FRIENDLY PACKETS)	METABOLISM MEAL REPLACEMENT SHAKE: 1½ SCOOPS	PEAR AND ¼ CUP RAW PISTACHIOS	RAINBOW CHICKEN AND VEGGIES

DAVID'S SUPER-SIMPLE SUPPORTED PLAN

avid works in law enforcement, and he is on the night shift, so he rarely gets to share a meal with his family and often finds himself in the kitchen in the early hours of the morning before sunrise, wolfing down whatever he can find for his so-called dinner. To his chagrin, David had gained 25 pounds during the first two years of his new job, and while he wanted to get in shape and back to a healthy weight, he found it extremely difficult. He was on the opposite schedule from his family, and when they were all awake at the same time, he wanted to be with them, not working out at the gym or worrying about following some diet plan.

I knew the Super-Simple Supported Plan would be perfect for David, whose Metabolic Intervention Score matched him with Meal Map B. I explained that he could easily bring his shakes and snacks to work with him, and if he preprepared a simple dinner, he would only have to warm it up when he came home early in the morning to eat something that supported his health goals.

Then I showed him how he could eat the same thing for every Part 1 day (the first three days of each week) and then the same thing for every Part 2 day (the second four days of each week). I helped him choose two meals he could cook with little effort and freeze so his meals would be ready for him. He shopped ahead and got a shaker bottle for his Metabolism Meal Replacement Shake, and he was ready to go.

Every evening he packed his portioned shake powder, two bottles of spring water, his two daily snacks, and his shake bottle, and took them to work with him. He told me he was never hungry because the shakes were so filling, and he felt like it was always time to eat again. Within fourteen days, David had lost 14 pounds, and decided to do the plan one more time to knock off the last 11 pounds.

Here is exactly what he did. Note that this meal map contains the two dinners David chose, but you could choose any Part 1 recipe and any Part 2 recipe to make ahead for your dinners. You could also make more than one dinner, if you have the time. Just be sure it coincides with the correct part and that you prepare it in the amount appropriate for Meal Map B.

(Note that weight, water, and exercise are not included in this sample meal map, but David tracked them, and you should, too, on your blank meal map following page 313.)

SUPER-SIMPLE SUPPORTED PLAN FOR MEAL MAP B: DAVID (Recipes start on page 123.)

	BREAKFAST	A.M. SNACK	LUNCH	P.M. SNACK	DINNER
PART 1 (MONDAY–WEDNESDAY)	METABOLISM MEAL REPLACEMENT SHAKE: 2 SCOOPS	APPLE	METABOLISM MEAL REPLACEMENT SHAKE: 2 SCOOPS	PEAR	LEMON-BASIL PORK WITH WILD RICE
PART 2 (THURSDAY–SUNDAY)	METABOLISM MEAL RE-PLACEMENT SHAKE: 2 SCOOPS	4 OUNCES NITRATE-FREE TURKEY DELI MEAT AND 10 OLIVES	METABOLISM MEAL REPLACEMENT SHAKE: 2 SCOOPS	4 OUNCES BACON CHIPS AND 1/4 CUP GUACAMOLE	SAUSAGE WITH ROASTED VEGGIES

SALLY'S SUPER-SIMPLE SUPPORTED PLAN

Sally has a big family—four kids ranging from ages four to thirteen. While Sally knew she needed to drop at least 50 pounds, she felt stuck because she had a family who loved to order pizza, pick up drive-through fast food, and snack on sweets. "And they're all skinny," she moaned. I explained that the reason she was the one having problems was because her metabolism needed repair, and that we could get that done together. She was motivated, but her biggest concern was her family. She knew they simply weren't in a place where they would be on board with the kind of foods she would be eating. "No problem," I told her. "The Super-Simple Supported Plan is for you."

We calculated Sally's Metabolic Intervention Score and determined that she needed Meal Map C, and I explained that with the supported plan, she could have easy shakes for breakfasts and lunches, portable snacks, and the same preprepared dinner every night for Part 1 and another one every night for Part 2. The rest of her family could get the food they wanted, while she focused on doing what she needed to do for herself. She was game, so we picked one Part 1 dinner and one Part 2 dinner. Because Meal Map C has a 3/4 split, she made six portions of the Part 1 dinner and eight portions of the Part 2 dinner. She put the meals for week 1 in the refrigerator, portioned into individual servings, and the meals for week 2 in the freezer. She was excited to start, and by the end of the fourteen days, she was down exactly 14 pounds. She was so inspired that she decided to do the plan again. And what's even better news is that her family was so curious about what she was doing, and so interested in the yummy home-cooked food she was eating, that they decided to help her do the regular plan the second time around. (But she still kept those shakes on hand for those extra-busy days.)

Here is exactly what she did. Note that this meal map contains the two dinners Sally chose, but you could choose any Part 1 recipe and any Part 2 recipe to make ahead for your dinners. You could also make more than one dinner, if you have the time. Just be sure it coincides with the correct part and you prepare it in the amount appropriate for Meal Map C.

(Note that weight, water, and exercise are not included in this sample meal map, but Sally tracked them, and you should, too, on your blank meal map following page 313.)

SUPER-SIMPLE SUPPORTED PLAN FOR MEAL MAP C: SALLY (Recipes start on page 123.)

	BREAKFAST	A.M. SNACK	LUNCH	P.M. SNACK	DINNER
PART 1 (MONDAY–WEDNESDAY)	METABOLISM MEAL REPLACEMENT SHAKE: 2 SCOOPS	1 CUP BLUEBERRIES	METABOLISM MEAL REPLACEMENT SHAKE: 2 SCOOPS	2 CUPS SLICED STRAWBERRIES	CHICKEN AND BLACK BEAN TACOS
PART 2 (THURSDAY–SUNDAY)	METABOLISM MEAL REPLACEMENT SHAKE: 2 SCOOPS	4 OUNCES NITRATE-FREE TURKEY DELI MEAT AND ¼ AVOCADO SLICED, WRAPPED IN LETTUCE LEAVES	METABOLISM MEAL REPLACEMENT SHAKE: 2 SCOOPS	4 OUNCES NITRATE-FREE BEEF JERKY, ¼ CUP HUMMUS, AND CELERY STICKS	GINGER-LIME SALMON

SUPPLEMENTARY MATERIAL

Here are all the at-a-glance and blank meal maps for the Metabolism Revolution plan, the Metabolism Revolution Food List, the Fast Metabolism 4 Life Meal Maps with exercise recommendations, and the FMD 4 Life Master Food List, for your easy reference.

Meal Map A (Metabolic Intervention Score 10 or greater)

Week One—Part 1

	A.M. WEIGHT	BREAKFAST	A.M. SNACK	LUNCH	P.M. SNACK	DINNER	OZ. OF WATER PER DAY	EXERCISE
MONDAY		RECIPE: OR 1 P: 1 V: 1 F: 1 G OR CC:	1 F:	RECIPE: OR 1 P: 2 V: 1 F:	1 F:	RECIPE: OR 1 P: 1 V: 1 CC:		
TUESDAY		RECIPE: OR 1 P: 1 V: 1 F: 1 G OR CC:	1 F:	RECIPE: OR 1 P: 2 V: 1 F:	1 F:	RECIPE: OR 1 P: 1 V: 1 CC:		
WEDNESDAY		RECIPE: OR 1 P: 1 V: 1 F: 1 G OR CC:	1 F:	RECIPE: OR 1 P: 2 V: 1 F:	1 F:	RECIPE: OR 1 P: 1 V: 1 CC:		
THURSDAY		RECIPE: OR 1 P: 1 V: 1 F: 1 G OR CC:	1 F:	RECIPE: OR 1 P: 2 V: 1 F:	1 F:	RECIPE: OR 1 P: 1 V: 1 CC:		

PART 1

KEY: P = Protein V = Veggie F = Fruit CC = Complex Carb G = Grain-Based Carb HF = Healthy Fat and Oils

Meal Map A

Week One—Part 2

	A.M. WEIGHT	BREAKFAST	A.M. SNACK	LUNCH	P.M. SNACK	DINNER	OZ. OF WATER PER DAY	EXERCISE
FRIDAY		RECIPE: OR 1 P: 1 V: 1 F:	1 F: 1 HF:	RECIPE: OR 1 P: 1 V: 1 HF:	1 P: 1 HF:	RECIPE: OR 1 P: 1 V: 1 HF:		
PART 2 SATURDAY		RECIPE: OR 1 P: 1 V: 1 F:	1 F: 1 HF:	RECIPE: OR 1 P: 1 V: 1 HF:	1 P: 1 HF:	RECIPE: OR 1 P: 1 V: 1 HF:		
SUNDAY		RECIPE: OR 1 P: 1 V: 1 F:	1 F: 1 HF:	RECIPE: OR 1 P: 1 V: 1 HF:	1 P: 1 HF:	RECIPE: OR 1 P: 1 V: 1 HF:		

KEY: P = Protein V = Veggie F = Fruit CC = Complex Carb G = Grain-Based Carb HF = Healthy Fat and Oils

Meal Map A (Metabolic Intervention Score 10 or greater)

Week Two—Part 1

	A.M. WEIGHT	BREAKFAST	A.M. SNACK	LUNCH	P.M. SNACK	DINNER	OZ. OF WATER PER DAY	EXERCISE
MONDAY		RECIPE: OR 1 P: 1 V: 1 F: 1 G OR CC:	1 F:	RECIPE: OR 1 P: 2 V: 1 F:	1 F:	RECIPE: OR 1 P: 1 V: 1 CC:		
TUESDAY		RECIPE: OR 1 P: 1 V: 1 F: 1 G OR CC:	1 F:	RECIPE: OR 1 P: 2 V: 1 F:	1 F:	RECIPE: OR 1 P: 1 V: 1 CC:		
WEDNESDAY		RECIPE: OR 1 P: 1 V: 1 F: 1 G OR CC:	1 F:	RECIPE: OR 1 P: 2 V: 1 F:	1 F:	RECIPE: OR 1 P: 1 V: 1 CC:		
THURSDAY		RECIPE: OR 1 P: 1 V: 1 F: 1 G OR CC:	1 F:	RECIPE: OR 1 P: 2 V: 1 F:	1 F:	RECIPE: OR 1 P: 1 V: 1 CC:		

PART 1

KEY: P = Protein V = Veggie F = Fruit CC = Complex Carb G = Grain-Based Carb HF = Healthy Fat and Oils

Meal Map A
Week Two—Part 2

	A.M. WEIGHT	BREAKFAST	A.M. SNACK	LUNCH	P.M. SNACK	DINNER	OZ. OF WATER PER DAY	EXERCISE
FRIDAY		RECIPE: OR 1 P: 1 V: 1 F:	1 F: 1 HF:	RECIPE: OR 1 P: 1 V: 1 HF:	1 P: 1 HF:	RECIPE: OR 1 P: 1 V: 1 HF:		
PART 2 SATURDAY		RECIPE: OR 1 P: 1 V: 1 F:	1 F: 1 HF:	RECIPE: OR 1 P: 1 V: 1 HF:	1 P: 1 HF:	RECIPE: OR 1 P: 1 V: 1 HF:		
SUNDAY		RECIPE: OR 1 P: 1 V: 1 F:	1 F: 1 HF:	RECIPE: OR 1 P: 1 V: 1 HF:	1 P: 1 HF:	RECIPE: OR 1 P: 1 V: 1 HF:		

KEY: P = Protein V = Veggie F = Fruit CC = Complex Carb G = Grain-Based Carb HF = Healthy Fat and Oils

Meal Map B (Metabolic Intervention Score 7 to 9)

Week One—Part 1

	A.M. WEIGHT	BREAKFAST	A.M. SNACK	LUNCH	P.M. SNACK	DINNER	OZ. OF WATER PER DAY	EXERCISE
MONDAY		RECIPE: OR 1 P: 2 V: 1 F: 1 G OR CC:	1 F:	RECIPE: OR 1 P: 2 V: 1 F:	1 F:	RECIPE: OR 1 P: 2 V: 1 CC:		
TUESDAY		RECIPE: OR 1 P: 2 V: 1 F: 1 G OR CC:	1 F:	RECIPE: OR 1 P: 2 V: 1 F:	1 F:	RECIPE: OR 1 P: 2 V: 1 CC:		
WEDNESDAY		RECIPE: OR 1 P: 2 V: 1 F: 1 G OR CC:	1 F:	RECIPE: OR 1 P: 2 V: 1 F:	1 F:	RECIPE: OR 1 P: 2 V: 1 CC:		

PART 1

KEY: P = Protein V = Veggie F = Fruit CC = Complex Carb G = Grain-Based Carb HF = Healthy Fat and Oils

Meal Map B
Week One—Part 2

	A.M. WEIGHT	BREAKFAST	A.M. SNACK	LUNCH	P.M. SNACK	DINNER	OZ. OF WATER PER DAY	EXERCISE
THURSDAY		RECIPE: OR 2 P: 1 V: 1 HF:	1 P: 1 HF:	RECIPE: OR 1 P: 2 V: 1 HF:	1 P: 1 HF:	RECIPE: OR 1 P: 2 V: 1 HF:		
FRIDAY		RECIPE: OR 2 P: 1 V: 1 HF:	1 P: 1 HF:	RECIPE: OR 1 P: 2 V: 1 HF:	1 P: 1 HF:	RECIPE: OR 1 P: 2 V: 1 HF:		
SATURDAY		RECIPE: OR 2 P: 1 V: 1 HF:	1 P: 1 HF:	RECIPE: OR 1 P: 2 V: 1 HF:	1 P: 1 HF:	RECIPE: OR 1 P: 2 V: 1 HF:		
SUNDAY		RECIPE: OR 2 P: 1 V: 1 HF:	1 P: 1 HF:	RECIPE: OR 1 P: 2 V: 1 HF:	1 P: 1 HF:	RECIPE: OR 1 P: 2 V: 1 HF:		

PART 2

KEY: P = Protein V = Veggie F = Fruit CC = Complex Carb G = Grain-Based Carb HF = Healthy Fat and Oils

Meal Map B (Metabolic Intervention Score 7 to 9)

Week Two—Part 1

	A.M. WEIGHT	BREAKFAST	A.M. SNACK	LUNCH	P.M. SNACK	DINNER	OZ. OF WATER PER DAY	EXERCISE
MONDAY		RECIPE: OR 1 P: 2 V: 1 F: 1 G OR CC:	1 F:	RECIPE: OR 1 P: 2 V: 1 F:	1 F:	RECIPE: OR 1 P: 2 V: 1 CC:		
PART 1 TUESDAY		RECIPE: OR 1 P: 2 V: 1 F: 1 G OR CC:	1 F:	RECIPE: OR 1 P: 2 V: 1 F:	1 F:	RECIPE: OR 1 P: 2 V: 1 CC:		
WEDNESDAY		RECIPE: OR 1 P: 2 V: 1 F: 1 G OR CC:	1 F:	RECIPE: OR 1 P: 2 V: 1 F:	1 F:	RECIPE: OR 1 P: 2 V: 1 CC:		

KEY: P = Protein V = Veggie F = Fruit CC = Complex Carb G = Grain-Based Carb HF = Healthy Fat and Oils

Week Two—Part 2

	A.M. WEIGHT	BREAKFAST	A.M. SNACK	LUNCH	P.M. SNACK	DINNER	OZ. OF WATER PER DAY	EXERCISE
THURSDAY		RECIPE: OR 2 P: 1 V: 1 HF:	1 P: 1 HF:	RECIPE: OR 1 P: 2 V: 1 HF:	1 P: 1 HF:	RECIPE: OR 1 P: 2 V: 1 HF:		
FRIDAY		RECIPE: OR 2 P: 1 V: 1 HF:	1 P: 1 HF:	RECIPE: OR 1 P: 2 V: 1 HF:	1 P: 1 HF:	RECIPE: OR 1 P: 2 V: 1 HF:		
SATURDAY		RECIPE: OR 2 P: 1 V: 1 HF:	1 P: 1 HF:	RECIPE: OR 1 P: 2 V: 1 HF:	1 P: 1 HF:	RECIPE: OR 1 P: 2 V: 1 HF:		
SUNDAY		RECIPE: OR 2 P: 1 V: 1 HF:	1 P: 1 HF:	RECIPE: OR 1 P: 2 V: 1 HF:	1 P: 1 HF:	RECIPE: OR 1 P: 2 V: 1 HF:		

KEY: P = Protein V = Veggie F = Fruit CC = Complex Carb G = Grain-Based Carb HF = Healthy Fat and Oils

Meal Map C (Metabolic Intervention Score 6 or less)

Week One—Part 1

	A.M. WEIGHT	BREAKFAST	A.M. SNACK	LUNCH	P.M. SNACK	DINNER	OZ. OF WATER PER DAY	EXERCISE
MONDAY		RECIPE: OR 2 P: 2 V: 1 F: 1 G OR CC:	1 F:	RECIPE: OR 1 P: 2 V: 2 F:	2 F:	RECIPE: OR 2 P: 2 V: 1 CC:		
PART 1 **TUESDAY**		RECIPE: OR 2 P: 2 V: 1 F: 1 G OR CC:	1 F:	RECIPE: OR 1 P: 2 V: 2 F:	2 F:	RECIPE: OR 2 P: 2 V: 1 CC:		
WEDNESDAY		RECIPE: OR 2 P: 2 V: 1 F: 1 G OR CC:	1 F:	RECIPE: OR 1 P: 2 V: 2 F:	2 F:	RECIPE: OR 2 P: 2 V: 1 CC:		

	A.M. WEIGHT	BREAKFAST	A.M. SNACK	LUNCH	P.M. SNACK	DINNER	OZ. OF WATER PER DAY	EXERCISE
THURSDAY		RECIPE: OR 2 P: 2 V: 1 HF:	1 P: 1 HF:	RECIPE: OR 2 P: 2 V: 1 HF:	1 P: 1 HF:	RECIPE: OR 2 P: 2 V: 1 HF:		
FRIDAY		RECIPE: OR 2 P: 2 V: 1 HF:	1 P: 1 HF:	RECIPE: OR 2 P: 2 V: 1 HF:	1 P: 1 HF:	RECIPE: OR 2 P: 2 V: 1 HF:		
PART 2 SATURDAY		RECIPE: OR 2 P: 2 V: 1 HF:	1 P: 1 HF:	RECIPE: OR 2 P: 2 V: 1 HF:	1 P: 1 HF:	RECIPE: OR 2 P: 2 V: 1 HF:		
SUNDAY		RECIPE: OR 2 P: 2 V: 1 HF:	1 P: 1 HF:	RECIPE: OR 2 P: 2 V: 1 HF:	1 P: 1 HF:	RECIPE: OR 2 P: 2 V: 1 HF:		

KEY: P = Protein V = Veggie F = Fruit CC = Complex Carb G = Grain-Based Carb HF = Healthy Fat and Oils

Meal Map C (Metabolic Intervention Score 6 or less)

Week Two—Part 1

	A.M. WEIGHT	BREAKFAST	A.M. SNACK	LUNCH	P.M. SNACK	DINNER	OZ. OF WATER PER DAY	EXERCISE
MONDAY		RECIPE: OR 2 P: 2 V: 1 F: 1 G OR CC:	1 F:	RECIPE: OR 1 P: 2 V: 2 F:	2 F:	RECIPE: OR 2 P: 2 V: 1 CC:		
PART 1 **TUESDAY**		RECIPE: OR 2 P: 2 V: 1 F: 1 G OR CC:	1 F:	RECIPE: OR 1 P: 2 V: 2 F:	2 F:	RECIPE: OR 2 P: 2 V: 1 CC:		
WEDNESDAY		RECIPE: OR 2 P: 2 V: 1 F: 1 G OR CC:	1 F:	RECIPE: OR 1 P: 2 V: 2 F:	2 F:	RECIPE: OR 2 P: 2 V: 1 CC:		

KEY: P = Protein V = Veggie F = Fruit CC = Complex Carb G = Grain-Based Carb HF = Healthy Fat and Oils

Meal Map 6
Week Two—Part 2

	A.M. WEIGHT	BREAKFAST	A.M. SNACK	LUNCH	P.M. SNACK	DINNER	OZ. OF WATER PER DAY	EXERCISE
THURSDAY		RECIPE: OR 2 P: 2 V: 1 HF:	1 P: 1 HF:	RECIPE: OR 2 P: 2 V: 1 HF:	1 P: 1 HF:	RECIPE: OR 2 P: 2 V: 1 HF:		
FRIDAY		RECIPE: OR 2 P: 2 V: 1 HF:	1 P: 1 HF:	RECIPE: OR 2 P: 2 V: 1 HF:	1 P: 1 HF:	RECIPE: OR 2 P: 2 V: 1 HF:		
PART 2 SATURDAY		RECIPE: OR 2 P: 2 V: 1 HF:	1 P: 1 HF:	RECIPE: OR 2 P: 2 V: 1 HF:	1 P: 1 HF:	RECIPE: OR 2 P: 2 V: 1 HF:		
SUNDAY		RECIPE: OR 2 P: 2 V: 1 HF:	1 P: 1 HF:	RECIPE: OR 2 P: 2 V: 1 HF:	1 P: 1 HF:	RECIPE: OR 2 P: 2 V: 1 HF:		

KEY: P = Protein V = Veggie F = Fruit CC = Complex Carb G = Grain-Based Carb HF = Healthy Fat and Oils

METABOLISM REVOLUTION EXERCISE AT A GLANCE

Meal Map A Recommended Exercise

- *Cardio:* 3 or 4 times per week, to raise your heart rate to between 120 and 140 beats per minute for 20 to 35 minutes for each session.
- *Weights:* No weight lifting during the 14-day program.
- *Metabolic Intervention Exercises:* : Minimum of 1 time per week.

Meal Map B Recommended Exercise

- *Cardio:* 2 or 3 times per week, to raise your heart rate to between 120 and 140 beats per minute for 20 to 35 minutes for each session.
- *Weights:* 1 time per week, focusing on 3 major muscle groups for each session.
- *Metabolic Intervention Exercises:* Minimum of 1 time per week.

Meal Map C Recommended Exercise

- *Cardio:* 2 or 3 times per week, to raise your heart rate to between 120 and 140 beats per minute for 20 to 35 minutes for each session.
- *Weights:* 2 times per week, focusing on 3 major muscle groups for each session.
- *Metabolic Intervention Exercises:* Minimum of 2 times per week.

METABOLISM REVOLUTION FOOD LIST

FREE FOODS

These can be incorporated into any meal at any time in unlimited quantities.

100% monk fruit/lo han
100% pure stevia
Birch xylitol
Celery
Dried or fresh herbs and spices
Egg whites
Garlic
Ginger
Horseradish

Lemons
Limes
Mustard, pure (no additives)
Onions
Pepper: Black, red pepper flakes
Raw cacao powder
Sea salt
Vinegar, pure (no additives)

FRUITS: 1 CUP = 1 PORTION

These can be fresh or frozen, and served in combination.

Apples
Berries, all
Cherries
Grapefruit
Mangoes
Melons, all

Nectarines
Oranges
Peaches
Pears
Pineapple
Plums

VEGETABLES: 2 CUPS RAW / 1 CUP COOKED = 1 PORTION

These can be fresh or frozen; served raw or cooked; and served in combination.

Asparagus
Beets, all
Broccoli/Broccolini
Cabbage
Carrots
Cauliflower
Cucumbers
Green beans, yellow beans, wax beans

Mixed leafy greens and lettuces
Mushrooms, all
Onions, all
Peppers, all
Radishes
Squashes, all

NON-GRAIN-BASED COMPLEX CARBS: ½ CUP COOKED = 1 PORTION

Beans/legumes (except peanuts, green
  peas, or soy)
Quinoa

Sweet potato/yams
Wild rice

GRAINS: ½ CUP COOKED = 1 PORTION

Brown rice
Buckwheat
Kamut

Oats
Spelt

PROTEINS: 4 OUNCES RAW OR 2 EGGS = 1 PORTION

Organic, free-range, and antibiotic-free is preferred. Select nitrite-free, with no additives, sugars, or preservatives.

Beef
Buffalo
Chicken
Eggs, whole
Fish, wild-caught

Lamb
Pork
Shrimp
Turkey
Wild game

VEGETARIAN PROTEINS

Edamame, ¾ cup (shelled)
Legumes, ¾ cup cooked (such as lentils,
  black beans, white beans, refried
  beans, etc.—*no peanuts*)
Mushrooms, any type, 3 cups (raw)

Tempeh, 4 ounces raw (the only soy
  product allowed)

HEALTHY FAT

These can be served in combination.

Avocado, ¼ avocado
Hummus, ¼ cup
Nut and seed butters, from raw nuts and
  seeds only, 2 tablespoons
Nuts and seeds, raw only, ¼ cup
Oils: avocado, coconut, grapeseed,
  olive, safflower, sunflower, walnut oil,
  2 tablespoons
Olives, 8 to 10

Raw coconut meat, ¼ cup
Safflower oil mayonnaise, 2 tablespoons

FAST METABOLISM 4 LIFE HEALTHY NUTRITION AND EXERCISE PLAN TEMPLATE

BREAKFAST	A.M. SNACK	LUNCH	P.M. SNACK	DINNER	OPTIONAL EVENING SNACK	EXERCISE
FRUIT	VEGGIE	FAT/ PROTEIN	VEGGIE	FAT/ PROTEIN	VEGGIE	CARDIO (2X/WK)
FAT/ PROTEIN	FAT/ PROTEIN	VEGGIE	FAT/ PROTEIN	VEGGIE	FAT/ PROTEIN	WEIGHT LIFTING (2X/WK)
COMPLEX CARB		FRUIT		OPTIONAL COMPLEX CARB		MIE (1X/ WK)
VEGGIE						REST DAY (2X/WK)

FMD LIFE MASTER FOOD LIST

VEGETABLES:

1 serving = minimum 2 cups raw

Artichokes
Asparagus
Bamboo shoots
Beans, all types (green, yellow, wax, and legumes), except soy
Beets, all types
Broccoli, all types
Brussels sprouts
Cabbage, all types
Cactus
Carrots
Cauliflower
Celery, all types
Cucumbers, all types

Cultured/fermented veggies, all types
Eggplant
Fennel
Fiddleheads (coiled fern leaves)
Grape leaves
Hearts of palm
Jerusalem artichoke
Jicama
Kale
Kohlrabi
Leafy greens, all types (lettuces, spinach, kale, etc.)
Leeks
Mushrooms

Okra
Onions, all types
Parsnips
Peppers, all types
Radishes, all types
Rhubarb
Rutabaga
Sea vegetables/seaweeds, all types
Snow peas
Spinach

Spirulina
Sprouts, all types
Squash, all types
Sweet potatoes
Taro
Tomatillos
Tomatoes
Turnips, all types
Wheatgrass
Yucca

FRUITS (FRESH OR FROZEN):

1 serving = 1 to 1 ½ cups or pieces

Apples, all types
Apricots
Berries, all types
Cherimoya
Cherries
Dragon fruit
Figs, fresh only
Grapefruit
Guavas
Jackfruit
Kiwi
Kumquats
Lemons
Limes
Loquats
Lychees
Mangoes
Melons, all types
Nectarines

Oranges, all types
Papayas
Passion fruits
Peaches
Pears, all types
Persimmons
Pineapple
Plantains
Plums
Pluots
Pomegranates
Pomelo
Prickly pears
Quince
Star fruits
Tamarind
Ugli fruit
Watermelon

COMPLEX CARBS

1 serving = ¼ to ⅔ cup cooked, or 1 slice or piece

Amaranth

Barley, all types

Buckwheat

Einkorn

Farro

Flours made from all approved grains

Freekah

Kamut

Milks made from all approved grains
  (like oat milk)

Millet

Oats (old-fashioned, steel-cut)

Pasta made from all approved grains

Quinoa

Rice, all types except white

Rye

Sorghum

Spelt

Sprouted wheat

Tapioca

Teff

Wheat berries (sprouted)

ANIMAL PROTEIN

1 serving = 4 to 5 ounces, or 2 eggs

Beef

Buffalo

Chicken

Collagen

Cornish game hen

Crustaceans, all types

Cured lean meats, all types (nitrate-free)

Deli meats, all types (nitrate-free)

Eggs

Escargot

Fish, all types (wild-caught, raw,
  smoked, canned)

Frog legs

Gelatin

Jerky, all types (nitrate-free)

Lamb

Mollusks, all types

Organ meats, all types

Pork, all types

Rabbit

Turkey, all types

Wild game, all types

VEGETABLE PROTEIN

1 serving = ¼ to ½ cup cooked, protein powder according to package directions

Beans/legumes, all types except green
  peas, peanuts, and soy (although
  vegans who are at their ideal weight
  and not currently experiencing
  hormonal issues may choose
  to eat fermented soy only, on
  occasion—see more about soy on
  page 235)

Lentils, all types

Vegetable protein powders (such as
  from pea, brown rice, etc.—*not soy*)

HEALTHY FATS

Avocado, ¼ to ½
Cacao butter, 1 to 2 tablespoons
Coconut, fresh or dried (unsweetened),
    ¼ to ½ cup
Hummus), ¼ to ½ cup
Mayonnaise (avocado, olive, safflower,
    sunflower), 1 to 2 tablespoons
Oils (avocado, coconut, grapeseed,
    olive, sesame, sunflower, safflower),
    1 to 2 tablespoons

Olives, all types, 8 to 10
Raw nuts and seeds, all types (including
    raw nut butters, milks, cheeses, and
    yogurts), ¼ to ½ cup nuts or seeds;
    1 to 2 tablespoons nut butters

HERBS, SPICES, CONDIMENTS, AND MISCELLANEOUS FOODS

Serving size is unlimited

Agar
Arrowroot powder
Baking powder
Baking soda
Bragg Liquid Aminos
Brewer's yeast
Broth and stock, all types (homemade or
    no sugar)
Carob (unsweetened)
Chile paste
Coconut aminos
Coconut water
Coffee substitutes (Dandy Blend, Pero)
Cream of tartar
Herbs, all types
Extracts, natural, all types (alcohol-free)
Flavorings and infusions, natural, all
    types (alcohol-free)
Guar gum
Herbal teas (caffeine-free)
Hot sauce, all types (no sugar added)
Ketchup (no corn syrup or sugar added)
Liquid smoke
Maca powder
Mustard, all types
Nutritional yeast

Pepper
Pickles (no sugar added)
Raw cacao powder and nibs
Salsa
Sea salt
Spices, all types
Sweeteners, natural (birch-based xylitol,
    coconut sugar, pure maple syrup,
    molasses, 100% pure monk fruit/lo
    han, palm sugar, raw honey, 100%
    pure stevia)
Tamari
Vinegars, all types
Water chestnuts
Xanthan gum (non-corn based)
Zest/peels (citrus)

ACKNOWLEDGMENTS

t's hard to believe I am thanking people for what they have meant to me during the writing of my fifth book! I never imagined I would be in this place, and it is in large part due to the personal and professional support, love, and care I have been privileged to receive from so many corners of my complex and crazy life.

First of all, Alex Glass, my brilliant agent, has been my steadfast champion through this roller-coaster ride of book publishing, and I could never have achieved five books, not to mention so many other crucial aspects of my career, without him. Alex, you are a godsend and the best in the business.

I am indebted to Harper Wave for forging a new relationship with me and taking my vision further into the future. Karen Rinaldi, Hannah Robinson, Brian Perrin, and Yelena Nesbit, thank you for trusting me and running with this—your work will help my work save lives and change the world.

Eve Adamson, we've been on a long journey together and I feel so fortunate to have had you by my side throughout it all. Your wordsmithing makes every page better. Bob Marty, my public television guru, thank you for spearheading this significant piece of our outreach. Melanie Parish, thank you for your continued guidance, both personally and professionally. Marc Chaplin, my legal pillar, your guidance has been and will continue to be invaluable to my business and my life. To Leilani, John, Carol, Tim, Wendy, Hanna, Emily,

Marq, and the whole HPG Team, thank you for making my mission your mission. We are doing something very important, and you make it happen.

None of this would be possible without my community of clients, both in-person and virtual, including my readers and everyone who joins me online for our many inspirational ventures. I love how savvy you have become, and the way you bring that knowledge to every new person who comes into the fold. You are the reason I do what I do, and making your lives better makes my life better. Thank you for that.

Finally, thank you to my crazy beautiful family: My parents, my sisters and sister in-law, my outlaw brothers, my cherished nieces and nephews, my outrageously precious kids, and my husband, who is my rock and whose deep well of love feeds me daily and is never ending. I love you with everything I have.

INDEX

ABOUT THE AUTHOR

AYLIE POMROY is a candidate for a master's degree in public health from The George Washington University and is the founder and CEO of the Haylie Pomroy Group, which houses her clinical practice, membership website, and coaching services. She is Hollywood's top nutrition guru, and her celebrity clients include Jennifer Lopez, Robert Downey Jr., LL Cool J, Reese Witherspoon, Raquel Welch, and Cher, along with professional and Olympic athletes and corporate executives of Fortune 500 companies. Her four internationally bestselling books have been published in fourteen languages.

hayliepomroy.com

HAYLIE POMROY
Real food, real people, real change.

WAIT!
Before you do anything, go to my website and
BECOME A MEMBER TODAY!

You will find delicious recipes, super simple meal maps, accesss to our private Facebook page, and more!

HayliePomroy.com